Recovery Skills Manual

Recovery Skills Manual

An Implementation Guide
for Addiction Care

Paul H. Earley

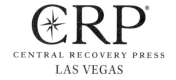

CENTRAL RECOVERY PRESS
LAS VEGAS

Central Recovery Press (CRP) is committed to publishing exceptional materials addressing addiction treatment, recovery, and behavioral healthcare topics.

For more information, visit www.centralrecoverypress.com.

© 2020 by Earley Consultancy, LLC

Publisher: Central Recovery Press
            3321 N. Buffalo Drive
            Las Vegas, NV 89129

25 24 23 22 21 20   1 2 3 4 5

ISBN: 978-1-949481-36-5 (paper)
978-1-949481-37-2 (e-book)

Photo of Paul Earley by Eric Bern of Eric Bern Studio. Used with permission.

Every attempt has been made to contact copyright holders. If copyright holders have not been properly acknowledged please contact us. Central Recovery Press will be happy to rectify the omission in future printings of this book.

Publisher's Note: This workbook is not an alternative to medical advice from your doctor or other professional healthcare provider. CRP books represent the experiences and opinions of their authors only. Every effort has been made to ensure that events, institutions, and statistics presented in our books as facts are accurate and up-to-date. To protect their privacy, the names of some of the people, places, and institutions in this workbook may have been changed.

Cover and interior design by Deb Tremper, Six Penny Graphics.

Contents

Welcome

This manual is a practical, step-by-step guide designed to help you implement RecoveryMind Training (RMT) in your outpatient practice (ASAM Level 1), IOP (Level 2.1), Partial Hospitalization (Level 2.5), or Residential program (Levels 3.1 to 3.7). It assumes you are already familiar with the basic concepts of RecoveryMind Training and can apply these concepts to the specific exercises this manual contains.

When you first introduce the techniques described here, it's important to remain faithful to the principles from *RecoveryMind Training* (the text). They have been carefully developed by experts in the field to ensure that each patient has the highest probability of success. As you become more familiar with each of the modules, I encourage you to provide me with feedback on changes and modifications you think might be helpful, since RecoveryMind Training is an evolving model of comprehensive treatment.

Before we begin, perhaps we should discuss terminology. I will use the terms *therapist* and *clinician* to refer to the individuals providing care. RecoveryMind Training does not define the credentials that a caregiver must have for a given task. I leave this up to licensing agencies, your training, your knowledge base, and your skill set. I will also use several terms for the individuals receiving treatment, using *patient* or *client* most often. I mean no offense if you use other terms for the people you work with. In the same vein, I will use the term *addiction* most often when referring to the illness we treat rather than *substance use disorder*. The reasons for using this label are complex. To learn more, please refer to the companion volume, *RecoveryMind Training*.

With these thoughts in mind, I would like to welcome you to treatment in the twenty-first century!

About This Manual

RecoveryMind Training divides recovery skills into six domains. The RMT domains are:

- Domain A: Containment
- Domain B: Recovery Basics
- Domain C: Emotional Resilience
- Domain D: Internal Narrative
- Domain E: Connectedness and Spirituality
- Domain F: Relapse Prevention Skills

This manual assumes you have read *RecoveryMind Training* and understand the principles in that book before you use the tools contained in this manual. You may also benefit from attending a training on RecoveryMind Training before you start. Contact me at paulearley.net for more information.

Each domain contains a group of skills. A patient practices a skill (if so assigned) until he or she develops the skill as defined and tracked in the Progress Assessment Form for each domain. As patients learn and practice these skills, they literally rewire the brain's neural pathways from the unconscious, reflexive addicted state (AddictBrain) to a balanced self-reflective state called RecoveryMind. Therapists who work in organized treatment use the following tools to structure the RecoveryMind Training process:

1. Assignment Groups
2. Skills Groups
3. Process Groups
4. Patient Worksheets
5. Progress Assessment Forms

Therapists in an outpatient practice may use groups as well, if so, they may use one or more of the group types 1, 2, and 3 above. If a therapist only works with clients individually, he or she fulfills more than one role, overseeing the work one minute and enrolling as an actor the next.

Studies point out that lecture-based training almost never modifies hardwired behaviors. Information is taught, but it is best followed by practice through role-play. Compare these two scenarios:

1. You tell your client, "You should not spend time with friends who are drinking, especially if they are intoxicated."

2. You first tell your client, "You should not spend time with friends who are drinking, especially if they are intoxicated." This is followed by, "Your good friend Amy, who goes with you to that club you like . . . What was its name? Yes, *The Inferno*. Stand up. I will play Amy. We are in *The Inferno*" The therapist talks a bit louder, gently taps her client's shoulder and says in a slight drawl that mimics early intoxication, "Oh come on have just one drink with me to celebrate." The client may correct the tone and delivery that Amy would adopt; if so the statement is repeated. Then the therapist falls out of role, subtly moves to one side a bit and asks, "What did that feel like?"

In the first case, your client learns a fact. In the second, he or she experiences the reality of that fact. Even if the role-play is quick and inaccurate, your client will experience a bit of the visceral experience of previous danger. You may choose to continue the role-play, having your client say, "No I have decided that I cannot drink alcohol . . . and furthermore, I should not be here." You may gently suggest he walks out the office door, shutting it firmly as he leaves.

If you have the luxury of working with many patients in a group setting, you probably already know how profound good therapy experiences can be for your clients. RecoveryMind Training asserts that skills that promote recovery are instilled through procedural learning (experiencing and moving) and not semantic memory (acquisition of facts).[1,2]

RecoveryMind Training uses lectures sparingly; therapy most often occurs in Skills Groups where the leader provides a short orientation to the tasks of that group. The orientation may be followed by limited participant discussion. The central therapeutic mode in Skills Groups is role-play or interactive practice, using the techniques derived from psychodrama[3,4] and PBSP psychomotor therapy.[5,6]

RecoveryMind Training defines three distinct types of group work. Each group type has distinctly different goals and flow of work. When beginning a group session, the therapist should clearly demarcate the group type to prevent confusion. At the beginning, a staff member or a patient says, "Welcome to Process (or Assignment or Skill) Group." This establishes the type of group being conducted and its purpose, thereby setting the tone and expectations for all members.

The first group type is the Assignment Group. Not surprisingly, Assignment Groups manage patient assignments. In an Assignment Group, patients who have tasks to complete (usually from completed worksheets) "bid for time" at the start of the group. The leader then prioritizes his or her agenda with the bids and tightly controls which patients will complete an assignment in each group.

Individual patients are directed to the next assignment at the start of the group *("David, if you are ready, you will present your Three by Five. Maria will you have your Addiction Life History ready by next Tuesday?").* Next, the leader has patients who have completed assignments read and discuss them in this group. Remember, Assignment Group is not a Process Group, but it does slide into group process a bit during assignment feedback and discussion.

In contrast, at the start of a Skills Group the leader announces a particular recovery skill, providing a short introduction to that skill. The leader describes the skill, role-plays it with one patient (called a *protagonist*, a term borrowed from psychodrama therapy) and then the entire group discusses the experience. The skill is repeated with additional protagonists as time permits.

Of the three types of groups, Process Group is the most unstructured. The group follows its own here-and-now process. Many therapists find it helpful to begin Process Group with a moment of mindfulness or centering. If the Process Group has new members, group rules and expectations are read. Otherwise, the therapist follows the moment of centering with utter silence. Patients begin when the group anxiety builds, often erupting when a patient says, "Well, I have something I need to talk about."

Appendix A has an in-depth discussion of about these group types. Example guidelines and rules for Process Group appear in Appendix B.

Regardless of whether the client is in outpatient therapy or in a residential program, it is best to review progress from time to time. This is accomplished by using a Progress Assessment Form for that domain. Once a patient completes the self-assessment portion of the form, the therapist completes his or her evaluation using the same items on the same form. The therapist reviews the Progress Assessment Form with the patient in an individual session. Using this system, the patient and the therapist (or the program) clarifies the amount of progress the patient has made and generates consensus—patients know what they need to work on, and staff know how the patient sees him- or herself. You can find Progress Assessment Forms at the end of each domain in this manual.

Patients may work on assignments in one (or possibly two) domains at the same time. They may spend more time on one particular domain or another, depending upon their particular needs. However, patients who suffer from attentional or cognitive problems may need to only work on assignments in one particular domain to prevent confusion.

This manual provides instructions for the therapist (for Skills Groups) and worksheets for the client in every domain. When you assign a worksheet, be sure to provide the entire worksheet to the client (including the introduction and instructions). Some clients may need additional supervision to complete a worksheet; they are rich experiences that warrant your careful attention to ensure a successful completion. Also, this manual will only cover the first five steps of Alcoholics Anonymous (AA) and Narcotics Anonymous (NA). Work on the remaining steps should continue with a sponsor at a point in time when the client is ready for continued step work.

The Progress Assessment Form for each domain has been carefully designed to ensure the client and the treatment team are clear about what progress has been made and what remains. This means that one form is passed back and forth several times between the client and staff (or therapist). Some treatment programs or therapists give the patient the Progress Assessment Form for those domain(s) to the client on a pretimed schedule—say at the end of the week. Other therapists may use give the client the relevant Progress Assessment Form(s) after a reasonable amount of assignments is completed. The client uses the form(s) to make a careful self-assessment of his or her status. Then the therapist (in a solo therapy practice) or the treatment team (in an organized treatment center) reviews the form. Once complete, it is reviewed with the client or patient. In this way, the patient is clear about progress and goals. The same form can be returned to the client two more times (if needed) for another round of self- and staff-assessment. This process highlights change, provides encouragement, and highlights accomplishments in RecoveryMind Training skills.

Feeling Overwhelmed?

The treatment process outlined in this manual may feel like it is quite a lot. It is. It has been designed that way. However, no single patient is expected to complete everything in this treatment manual. Patients who are being cared for in less intense levels (e.g., ASAM Level 2.1[7]) may only complete work in Domains A and B during their initial phase of treatment. Patients moving through a continuum from ASAM Levels 3.5 to 2.1 may complete work in Domains A through E over many weeks of tapering care. Keep in mind that addiction treatment is a multi-year process; it can take all this time to unwind the maladaptive learning induced by the disease. If a patient remains stable, you keep moving forward with work in this manual, dictated by patient needs.

If, for example, a client has a brief relapse when six months into recovery, the first thing to do is stabilize the illness. This may be achieved by changing addiction medications (buprenorphine, naltrexone, disulfiram, topiramate, and the like), a contractual commitment to family or therapist, or a brief stabilization at a higher level of care. The therapist reviews the relapse in detail and may change the focus of treatment to respond to the relapse. Work may begin in Domain F (Relapse Prevention Skills), for example, if the client and therapist discover that more relapse prevention skills are needed.

Let's consider the client Maria introduced above. She arrives in your office or treatment center with a firm understanding and acceptance of twelve-step recovery, but she is only partially stable in her recovery. In such a case there is no need to consider all (or at times any) assignment in Domain B (Recovery Basics). During the initial reassessment and treatment team review, staff decide which assignments will be most helpful to Maria in her current recovery path. If Maria has had repeated relapses trying to manage troubling emotions, for example, she would focus on Domain C.

In the case of a relapse, it is helpful to have the patient complete one or more Progress Assessment Form(s), once his or her immediate circumstances stabilize, to assess additional needs. RecoveryMind Training views a return to substance use (or even its antecedents) as an opportunity to reconsider the acquisition of additional recovery skills that will strengthen the patient's recovery program.

A Brief Note about the Structure of This Manual

You have just completed the introductory section of this manual. Each of remaining chapters covers one of the six domains of RecoveryMind Training. Each chapter begins with a refresher on the basic concepts underlying the respective domain. It then goes on to:

1. teach you how to train specific skills within that domain;
2. describe how to use assignments within that domain;
3. provide a self-assessment tool for that domain.

Remember that RecoveryMind Training is not an exhaustive compendium of mental health services. Rather, it focuses on a group of tools designed to help patients or clients attain remission from addiction. Clients should be evaluated for mood and anxiety disorders, the consequences of trauma, personality issues, and their need for a wide variety of Recovery Support Services (see Appendix C for a list of common Recovery Support Services). This does not mean that the effects of work in a given domain will not help conditions besides addiction, however. Work in Domain C, for example can help with mood disorders, personality difficulties, and troubles with anxiety.

About This Manual Notes

1. W. T. Maddox, and F. G. Ashby. "Dissociating Explicit and Procedural-Learning Based Systems of Perceptual Category Learning." *Behav Processes* 66, no. 3 (2004): 309-32.

2. R. Bourtchouladze. *Memories Are Made of This*. London: Phoenix Press, 2002.

3. A. Blatner. *Acting-In: Practical Applications of Psychodramatic Methods*. Third ed.: Springer Publishing Company, 1996.

4. N. P. F. Kellermann. *Focus on Psychodrama: The Therapeutic Aspects of Psychodrama*. Jessica Kingsley, 1992.

5. G. Slaninová, and P. Pidimová. "Pesso Boyden System Psychomotor as a Method of Work with Battered Victims." *Procedia - Social and Behavioral Sciences* 112 (2014): 387-94.

6. A. Pesso, and J. Crandell. *Moving Psychotherapy: Theory and Application of Pesso System/Psychomotor*. Cambridge: Brookline Books, 1991.

7. American Society of Addiction Medicine. *The ASAM Criteria: Treatment Criteria for Addictive, Substance-Related and Co-Occurring Disorders*. Edited by David Mee-Lee. Third ed. Carson City, Nevada: The Change Companies, 2013.

Domain A: Containment

Skills Groups, Assignments, Worksheets, and the Progress Assessment Forms

Chapter Overview

To understand containment requires understanding the psychological concept of "locus of control." The concept of locus of control was developed by one of the preeminent psychologists of the twentieth century, Julian Rotter.[1] At the extremes, individuals either have an internal locus of control or rely strictly on an external locus of control. RecoveryMind Training asserts that individuals with substance use disorders, by definition, lack internal controls over their substance use, which leads to loss of control. Therefore, containment is used to achieve abstinence. I use external containment when a patient has a complete loss of control and maintain the containment until internalized recovery occurs.

Containment alone does not produce or ensure recovery, but it does allow one to start the journey. Said another way, abstinence is a prerequisite for recovery (sobriety). If there is failure to contain addictive behaviors, progress **halts** in all other areas of treatment.[2] Containment is also used to provide a needed break during periods where AddictBrain swamps and overrides RecoveryMind.

It is quite normal and acceptable for commitment to abstinence and recovery to wax and wane, especially early in the process. As ambivalence improves, patients take more ownership of past behaviors and of their need for self-care. Sometimes this is referred to as "internalizing recovery." The patient's locus of control shifts from external to partially internalized though the course of recovery.

One important treatment task is to help clients recognize their ambivalence about recovery and to accept external containment as a helpful tool to employ, most frequently at first and from time to time along the course of a successful sobriety. Complete acceptance in not a requirement; patients may intellectually accept the need for ongoing urine drug screens, for example, and simultaneously ill at ease with the containment these provide.

I engage their reflective RecoveryMind, asking it to consider the importance of using containment to control AddictBrain, while simultaneously validating recovery ambivalence. No one is 100 percent committed to recovery 100 percent of the time. In fact, asking your patients or clients for perfection is a formula for disaster. Programs that continue to provide containment for addiction by continuing medications, cataloging support group attendance, obtaining drug screens, and monitoring ongoing therapy show remarkable long-term outcomes.[3-5]

It is just as critical to emphasize that AddictBrain thinking never dies. Individuals with decades of recovery continue to have moments where they consider a return to drinking or other drug use. During these times, the recovering individual can use cognitive behavioral techniques (thought-based containment) to reorient his thinking. Failing this, he can dust off a past containment vehicle and use it during times of danger.

RecoveryMind Training defines four types of containment:

1. **Physical:** Physical containment practices include geographical, structural, or taken to the extreme, locks on doors that stop access to substance use or process addictions.

2. **Social:** Social containment uses the power of a group to modify behavior and prevent relapse.

3. **Contractual:** Contractual containment is also known as contingency contracting or contingency management (CM).[6-8] Contractual Containment uses verbal or written contracts designed to use operant conditioning to shape pro-recovery behaviors. The contract outlines how the behavior shaping occurs through positive or negative reinforcement. An example of a negative reinforcement is when an adolescent is permitted to drive the family car as long as he or she has negative drug screens. The rate of a behavior increases because an adverse event (losing the ability to drive) is prevented. This type of negative reinforcement ranges from the above driving restriction all the way to spending time in jail for a positive urine screen. Carefully constructed, contingency management can be the centerpiece of containment after an individual begins his or her recovery journey.

4. **Biological:** Biological containment uses medications that interfere with the effect of a drug or change brain chemistry to assist with abstinence. For example, disulfiram may prove helpful in the motivated individual who is recovering from an alcohol use disorder. Buprenorphine, by decreasing craving and partially blocking the opioid effect, produces biological containment. Naltrexone blocks the effects of opioids and alters the response to alcohol in the recovering individual.

Introduction to Skills, Assignments, and Assessment Forms

Each subsequent chapter in this manual describes Skills Groups, the assigned Worksheet Assignments, and the Progress Assessment Form. Domain A has five Skills Groups, the last of which is used later in the treatment course. Note than some of the worksheets used to teach these skills have a paired assignment to read aloud and discuss. Other worksheets are completed solely by the client and reviewed with a staff member or therapist.

Domain A Skills

A1) Introduction to Containment

A2) Types of Containment

A3) Recognizing AddictBrain

A4) Resistance to Containment

A5) Modifications in Containment over Time

Domain A Worksheets

A1) *Efforts to Control Worksheet*

A2) *Containment Desirability Worksheet*

A3) *Containment and Me Worksheet*

A4) *Changing Containment over Time Worksheet*

Domain A Tasks for Assignment Group

A1) The client completes the *Efforts to Control Worksheet*. If he or she has access to a group setting, the worksheet is read in an Assignment Group and is followed by group feedback. If the client is in individual therapy, it is read aloud and discussed with his or her therapist.

A2) Once a client's illness has been controlled for a period of time, he or she should complete the *Changing Containment over Time* (A4) *Worksheet*. This worksheet helps a patient and the therapist or team consider when and how containment is tapered.

In Domain A, as in every domain, there is one *Progress Assessment Form.*

Domain A: Skills Groups

Skills Group A1: Introduction to Containment

In this Skills Group, the leader explains the basic concepts behind locus of control. The leader provides examples of external and internal control loci, using everyday examples. Patients are then asked for examples of loci of control from their own past including early childhood. The leader normalizes loss of control (e.g., "Everyone eats too much from time to time . . ."). It is a normal human phenomenon. However, addiction is a disease that produces consistent, predictable, and devastating loss of control that leads to addiction's progressive downhill course.

Next, the leader describes how the locus of control will change with recovery, moving from a predominantly external locus of control in early abstinence to a largely internal locus of control in long-term, sustained recovery. It is important to emphasize that individuals in recovery never attain a pure internal locus of control, even with decades of sobriety. Several examples of this may prove helpful as well.

Patients are then encouraged to role-play different containment strategies. Physical, contractual, and social containment are easiest to role-play. This module can be combined with the module directly below.

Skills Group A2: Types of Containment

This Skills Group has the largest education component of the four. It follows the Introduction to Containment group. Leaders may want to start A2 within the same session as A1 and continue this group at another Skills Group period. Patients are taught about the four types of containment. The leader provides examples of each. Patients are asked to discuss the four types of containment and ask questions about the desirability and effectiveness of each. If questions are raised about each type of containment, especially if the question cannot be answered with a brief response, it is best for the leader to answer the question with a role-play. "Let's see what that would look like. Reggie, you play the protagonist and we will see where it leads." Participants should leave this group understanding the containment components that make up an enduring recovery plan.

During this group, staff introduce the importance of long-term urine drug screening as an element of contractual containment. Patients are encouraged to discuss their resistance to ongoing urine screens; the leader responds by patiently returning to the principles behind this ongoing care modality. Urine screens provide an external validation (patients can prove to family, work, licensing agencies, and legal entities that they remain abstinent from substances that are misused). Screens also provide a "speed bump" that slows down using thoughts, the individual with an addiction disorder knows that if he does use substances, he will have to deal with consequences right away. Cravings are also reduced in many individuals and to varying intensity as a screen makes substance use transparent,[9] this decreases speculation about substance use and its associated craving.

During this training module, patients are also introduced to the concept of contingency contracting. If further along in recovery, negative urine screens confirm that the current treatment plan is effectively containing the illness. Positive urine screens, on the other hand, indicate to the patient and staff that a revision in the current treatment plan is indicated. Once the patient has established a solid foundation, continuing drug screening with contingencies for positive screens ensure the best long-term prognosis.

Skills Group A3: Recognizing AddictBrain

When using RecoveryMind Training, I borrow role-playing techniques from psychodrama and psychomotor therapy techniques. During Skills Groups, the leader explains the purpose of experiential psychotherapy, focusing on how it induces a deeper understanding than lectures or conventional therapeutic techniques. For many patients, this Skills Group will represent the first time they have participated in experiential psychotherapy. Skills Group A3 is one opportunity to discuss the basics of this modality.

If you choose to discuss basics, the following definitions should be reviewed:
- The director (the group leader)
- The stage (the area of the group room dedicated to the role-playing experience)
- A scene (the portion of a group focused on one individual's experience)
- The protagonist (the member of the group who is at the center of the current scene)
- Auxiliaries or actors (other individuals on the stage in the current scene)
- The concept of "enrolling" and "disenrolling"
- The audience (those who are watching and do not have a specified role in the current scene)

It may prove helpful to repeat this information or parts of this information from time to time, especially when new members join.

In Skills Group A3, the leader describes how AddictBrain hijacks an individual who suffers from addiction. This occurs in four specific ways:
- By strongly rewarding addiction-related behaviors
- By motivating an individual to seek out and continue substance use or behavioral addictions
- By instilling automatic learned responses that override conscious choice
- By reorganizing reality to make self-destructive addiction-related behaviors make sense to the afflicted individual

In this role-play, the director asks the group for a volunteer. The volunteer is the protagonist. He or she comes up on the stage and describes a scene from the past where he or she might have engaged in using behavior. It is best if this scene has elements of conflict (such as when the protagonist made an initial decision not to drink at a party but wound up doing so anyway).

The protagonist then selects members of the group to role-play each of the auxiliary functions of AddictBrain. The director teaches each auxiliary about his or her role and helps him or her practice auxiliary responses. In doing so, you are taking internal and poorly recognized brain processes and making them explicit and obvious within the protagonist's chosen scene. The director instructs the protagonist to start the scene at a slowed pace. For example, the protagonist may approach a table where drinks are served; each auxiliary then acts or speaks his or her role. For example, assume the protagonist is in front of a table on which the director establishes there are imaginary drinks. The scene continues as follows:

- The actor who is the voice of minimization might say, "One drink won't hurt"
- A second actor who is the voice promising reward might say, "It would feel so good to feel that feeling again."
- A third actor, who is role-playing "automatic behavior," might gently grab the protagonist's arm (after first requesting permission) and moving the hand to a table where invisible drinks are said to be present.
- And maybe the voice of denial might say something like, "You only drink because you are awkward in social situations."

The director closely watches the protagonist. If a statement rings true, she asks, "What are you feeling?" If a statement is rejected as incorrect, the leader queries the protagonist, saying, "That was not quite right, was it? Can you tell this auxiliary what to say (or do)?" The auxiliaries modify behaviors and words to more accurately depict the historical (or potential future) scene. It is much more important to have a few actions in this Skills Group deeply validated than to run through the whole scene. Take your time.

The audience is encouraged to watch and consider the current scene carefully. Save questions for the end of the role-play if possible. If an audience member has a question that the director senses is important, he or she explicitly instructs all actors on the stage to stop and temporarily come out of their assigned roles. Such interruptions should be carefully controlled to ensure that the protagonist and actors remain true to the scene at hand.

At the conclusion of a given scene, the actors disenroll and return to the group circle. At this point, any member present can share what he or she witnessed, felt, or learned. Emotional sharing is encouraged strongly above analytic comments. If time permits, the director encourages a second or third scene to be played out with a new protagonist followed by group sharing.

Skills Group A4: Resistance to Containment

Containment is a tool that is used primarily at the start of treatment to ensure abstinence. Patients' responses to containment vary across a wide continuum. At one extreme, a patient may balk or revolt from the simplest attempts to keep her safe from her disease. An example of this is the patient who elopes from a detoxification facility. At the other end of the spectrum, you may have a patient who has intense dependent characteristics who adopts all external controls readily, jailing herself in her own abstinence. Most patients are somewhere between these two extremes. In all cases containment needs should be tailored to the individual and evolve over time.

This Skills Group reviews the natural resistances to containment. The group starts with a general statement such as "No one likes to be told what to do." The module then reviews information from previous modules about the importance of containment as a tool for abstinence. Having established the natural tendency to eschew containment, the brief introductory lecture moves on to explore the types and qualities of this resistance. RecoveryMind Training states that there are two basic categories of containment resistance: The first comes from AddictBrain and occurs in all patients; the second type of resistance to containment arises from personality issues having to do with control. Patient resistance to containment should be discussed though open, nonjudgmental dialog.

To help patients visualize the resistance created by AddictBrain, the leader briefly describes how addictive drug use changes brain physiology. Addiction trains the brain, creating modifications to brain circuits once addiction takes hold. This entrainment is what I refer to as "AddictBrain." Once AddictBrain thinking is established, its primary goal is self-survival. It alters the thoughts, behaviors, and beliefs in those with substance use disorders. When a well-meaning treatment center introduces techniques designed to defeat it, AddictBrain quickly reacts with faultfinding and derision. It makes up interesting (and at times absurdist) responses such as "I want my addiction to heal naturally on its own." The leader might point out the irrationality of such arguments with examples from other areas of medicine (such as going to the doctor with a broken arm and saying, "I want to do this on my own."). If we truly accept the biological nature of addiction, it is simply common sense to pull out all the tools that will ensure a sustainable recovery. Nonetheless, nearly every patient will exhibit resistance to commitment. As clinicians, our job is to create awareness of this resistance, to pull it from the reactive and behavioral level to the reflective and contemplative level. Worksheet A3 helps patients explore their own life events that contribute to problems accepting needed outside help. Expanding on this worksheet in Skills Group A3, the leader may role-play voices that embody containment types along with voices for AddictBrain and RecoveryMind for the protagonist.

Resistance to addiction containment arises in individuals who, for a variety of reasons, have issues with trust. Examples of possible antecedents of this resistance would be individuals with

- Past physical, sexual, or emotional trauma;
- Overbearing parental domination or control;
- Untrustworthy parental figures;
- Neglectful parental figures, such that they had to raise themselves;
- Loss of parental figures through divorce, death, or abandonment;
- An abusive or controlling marital situation;
- Ongoing conflict between a parental figure and an adolescent or a failure to launch young adult behaviors;
- Narcissistic entitlement;
- An antisocial personality or characteristics;
- Avoidant disorders or social phobia.

As you can see, this list covers a wide variety of conditions that have the potential to sabotage effective disease containment. The approach to each of these different conditions is varied. The treatment team should catalog a given patient's resistance, working to build buy-in through the process of treatment. During this group, each of these potential problem areas should be discussed. If the role-playing exercise described above is used, additional voices from the patient's past are brought into the room.

Patient sharing in this area is often lively and profound. Some of the content that arises from this Skills Group may spill over into Process Group.

Skills Group A5: Modifications in Containment over Time

This Skills Group is optional and is best reserved for patients in longer-term recovery.

Having one's addiction contained is not the same thing as addiction recovery. It is impractical and undesirable to use prolonged physical containment to ensure abstinence, for example. This would be tantamount to swapping the addiction jail with abstinence jail.

As a patient internalizes recovery skills over time, he or she normally requires less containment. When containment is not buttressed by recovery skills, however, true sobriety never occurs. If a patient requires containment on an ongoing basis, he or she is probably not mastering recovery skills. Many of us have seen individuals who take prescribed disulfiram for years without practice in needed recovery skills. They wind up relying exclusively on this drug for abstinence. The disulfiram is consumed faithfully for months, but one day they "forget" to take it. RecoveryMind Training considers this in a different light by the way, reframing the forgetful episode as active, unconscious, or partly conscious sabotage by AddictBrain. Relapse occurs shortly thereafter.

One of the most difficult skills to learn in recovery is when external control can be safely reduced without risking relapse. In early treatment, the therapist or treatment center staff may be the best judge of when someone's containment should be modified. However, as an individual matures into his or her recovery, he or she increases insight into his or her own containment needs, adapting them to his or her stress, emotional state, and living situation.

The final Skills Group and worksheet in Domain A is designed to help patients self-regulate containment needs. At the start of this teaching module, the leader may ask a question such as "How do you know when you need more or less help staying sober?" Members of the group might offer suggestions that would include external as well as internal factors threatening relapse. Such discussion begins the process of relapse prevention training (Domain F). If the group is timid or new to treatment, this discussion will fall silent quickly. If this is the case, the leader might propose one of the following scenarios for discussion.

> *Scenario #1: Frank is attending an evening intensive outpatient program for his opioid dependence disorder. He was tired of "going nowhere" and has identified his addiction as a major contributor to his life problems. He begins treatment with enthusiasm and dives into RecoveryMind Training. At first, his old friends leave him alone. However, after five weeks, several of them show up at his house one Saturday afternoon, obviously high. After spending time with them, Frank is left feeling confused and ambivalent about his recovery.*
>
> - *Which of Frank's feelings might indicate he needs a change in containment?*
> - *Play out several scenarios that might occur in Frank's head after his friends leave. Which of these might indicate he needs a change in containment?*
> - *Play out several follow-up situations where Frank spends time with his using friends. Which of them might indicate that he needs a change in containment? Which of them would indicate that his recovery remains safe? Are there any actions at this point that might indicate he might do fine with less containment?*
>
> *Scenario #2: Jane returns home from residential treatment. At home, her husband and two young children have left the household fall into disarray. Jane's continued therapy plan states she will attend five AA meetings per week at first. She contracted to go to individual therapy and see her addiction medicine physician monthly. She agreed to modify her*

disease containment contract after discussion with her therapist and addiction medicine physician. Returning home, she finds the household in chaos.

- *Assume Jane does follow her contract exactly for the first two months. What feelings, behaviors, and situations in the home would indicate that Jane is safe to modify her containment, if any?*
- *Assume she continues to attend twelve-step meetings and therapy but is becoming increasingly frustrated with the chaos at home. When she first arrived home, her husband had stopped drinking but now a six-pack of beer regularly sits in the refrigerator. What, if anything, should Jane do about her containment now?*

Domain A: Containment Worksheets

Overview of Worksheets

Teaching patients about containment is easy. Implementing it proves more difficult. The worksheets in Domain A are designed to deepen a patient's understanding about disease containment. These worksheets will also shift a patient from seeing containment as "Containment of My Bad Self" to what it truly is—containing AddictBrain.

Containment is defined as "any pre-established relapse prevention technique that relies upon an external locus of control." Using the RecoveryMind Training principle, "To know it you must name it," patients are taught to label each aspect of their containment in every phase of treatment.

Four worksheets are available for Domain A:

1. *Efforts to Control* worksheet
2. *Containment Type Desirability* worksheet
3. *Containment and Me* worksheet
4. *Changing Containment over Time* worksheet

Worksheet #1 (*Efforts to Control*) only needs to be assigned to individuals who are struggling with accepting that addiction is controlling them. When assigned, a patient fills out the worksheet and presents it to his therapist or in Assignment Group. While I recommend all clients fill out this worksheet, if they do not have any issues in this area, then they can skip it and go to Worksheet #2.

Worksheet #2 (*Containment Desirability*) allows a patient to consider the types of containment and rank the acceptability of each. Upon review, he or she may benefit from reading his or her responses to Worksheet #2 aloud, but this is a less common Assignment Group task.

Worksheet #3 (*Containment and Me*) explores dynamic resistances to containment that often predate the development of one's addictive disease. These cover past traumas, childhood dynamics, or adult distress produced by oppressive marriages or work situations. Patients with these types of histories are naturally resistant to containment—it feels like their therapist or treatment team is heaping more coercion on an already oppressed soul. The results of Worksheet #3 should be reviewed individually with the patient and discussed in a Process Group.

Worksheet #4 (*Changing Containment over Time*) might be assigned to individuals who have already accepted their need for containment, have reviewed and accepted reasonable containment structures for the future, and have either few resistances to containment or exhibit good psychological insight to these resistances. Shorter-term treatment programs might not have time to cover this worksheet—it is best reserved for continuing care. It should not be assigned to those who have not accepted the need for containment or who are convinced they will get better using a "quick fix."

Worksheet A1: Efforts to Control

Briefly describe five instances in your past where you committed to yourself or another person to modify your addiction-related behaviors, and you failed. Then describe what happened.

Event and Description	R
Event: _____ What Happened: _____ _____ _____ _____ _____ _____	
Event: _____ What Happened: _____ _____ _____ _____ _____ _____	
Event: _____ What Happened: _____ _____ _____ _____ _____ _____	

Event and Description	R
Event: _____ What Happened: _____ _____ _____ _____ _____	
Event: _____ What Happened: _____ _____ _____ _____ _____ _____	

Now go back and place a #1 in the column to the right of the event that was most painful. Continue to rate each event in this manner, #1 being the most problematic or hurtful to you or others, and #5, the least.

How have you been successful in controlling your addiction illness?

_____

_____

_____

_____

_____

How have you not been successful?

_____

_____

_____

_____

_____

_____

Worksheet A2: Containment Desirability

Review this list of possible disease containment techniques. As you do so, remember that all recovering individuals need containment to attain and maintain abstinence. This need will decrease over time but not as quickly as you might like.

Rate each of these containment techniques on a scale of 1 to 5, five being the most desirable, and one being the least desirable. Put this number in the Like/Dislike column on the left. If a given containment technique is not applicable to you, put N/A in column ②, the Like/Dislike column. Then go back and carefully consider which of these types of containment you feel will be most effective or helpful, *regardless of how much you might like or dislike them*. Rate them on a scale of 1 to 5, five being the most helpful and one being the least helpful. Put you rating in column ③.

①	② Like / Dislike	③ Will Be the Most Effective	④ Containment Type	⑤ Description
			Physical	Locked detox unit
				Residential treatment
				Treatment in a remote location
				Removing alcohol and other addictive substances from the household
				Use of a GPS to decrease access to high-risk locations
				Computer software that prevents access to sex and gambling sites (for gambling and sexual dependence)
				Withholding access to an automobile or other transportation
			Social	Supportive living with daily check in for accountability
				Supportive living with rules that limit outside contact
				Living in a therapeutic community
				Daily contact with a sponsor who directs your actions
				Daily contact with a sponsor who only offers advice
			Contractual	Random urine, hair, and/or blood screening

①	② Like / Dislike	③ Will Be the Most Effective	④ Containment Type	⑤ Description
			Contractual (continued)	Contract with a treatment center that outlines your future actions in case of imminent or actual relapse
				Signed, written contract
				Verbal agreement
				Written and signed contract with workplace, employer, spouse, or regulatory agency that outlines mandated actions in case of imminent or actual relapse
				Verbal agreement with workplace, employer, spouse, or regulatory agency that outlines mandated actions in case of imminent or actual relapse
				Using a recovery diary to record therapy appointments, twelve-step meeting attendance, and visits with sponsor
			Biological	Medications that cause a negative reaction such as disulfiram for alcohol use disorder
				Medications that decrease craving and prevent withdrawal, such as buprenorphine for opioid addiction
				Medications that prevent drugs from having the desired effect such as naltrexone for opioid addiction
			Other	Describe any other ideas around containment you think might help below

Now go back through this list and put a checkmark in column ① next to the containment techniques that you think you should use in early recovery, balancing out how effective they might be with how acceptable they would be for you to use.

Discuss your choices with your therapist or in Assignment Group.

Worksheet A3: Containment and Me

Many people arrive in addiction treatment with earlier life experiences that get in the way of accepting help. If you grew up with a parent who was always controlling your behavior, for example, it might be difficult when your therapist tells you what to do or even suggests a different plan to you. Many aspects of addiction recovery feel awkward or difficult at first. You may tell yourself to go along with the treatment but find yourself resisting external direction.

This is important: **When AddictBrain takes over, it exaggerates resistances created in your past.** After all, if you resist treatment, AddictBrain eventually gets its way. It will use whatever it can to win. The purpose of this worksheet is to unearth past tendencies to resist external direction, even if it might save your life. As you fill out this form, remember that almost everyone has some oppositional tendencies. It's normal. The most important thing in RecoveryMind Training is to recognize your oppositional characteristics and prevent AddictBrain from using them against you.

Unlike many of the worksheets, you may want to review your answers with your therapist or a staff member prior to discussion in Assignment Group. This should make it easier to be forthcoming about past hurts and trauma.

Question 1: Go through the list below, marking items that apply to you by placing a check mark in column ①. There are open slots at the end of this worksheet where you can enter other feelings or experiences that have led to mistrust, defiant behavior, or be unwilling to accept external direction. Then go through the list a second time and rate intensity or importance of the checked items in column ②. Use a scale of 1 to 5, five being the most powerful, and one the least powerful in preventing you from accepting external direction in your recovery and addiction containment.

①	② Rank 1 to 5	③ Event, repeated event, personality characteristic, or feeling
		Past or present physical trauma or abuse
		Past or present emotional trauma or abuse
		Past or present sexual trauma or abuse
		Trauma related to military service
		Trauma related to violence in your home or neighborhood
		House arrest as a juvenile or adult
		Past incarceration or probation
		Overbearing parental domination or control
		Untrustworthy parental figures
		Neglect, had to raise myself
		Loss of parental figures through divorce, death, or abandonment
		Abusive or controlling marriage or partnership
		Severe conflict between you and a parent or parental figure
		Feeling controlled because you have not been able to move away from your family as a young adult
		A tendency to believe you are better than others or know more than they do, so rules often seem silly
		A tendency to believe that the rules do not apply to you, or you can manipulate others to allow you to do what you would like
		Difficulties with social situations or people who are severe enough that you isolate or avoid contact with others

Question 2: Next, using the above question as a guide, describe how these past events might make it difficult to accept the external control that is part of treatment (showing up for therapy sessions or groups, showing up late, having to give drug screens, and the like).

_____

_____

_____

_____

_____

Question 3: Finally, write out your thoughts as to what you can do to accept guidance and addiction containment as a necessary tool for your recovery.

_____

_____

_____

_____

_____

Worksheet A4: Changing Containment Over Time

Please do not work on this worksheet until you have sufficient time in recovery.

Place a checkmark in column ① for each of the behaviors that might get in the way of your decision to change your containment. Then, go through the list a second time and rank the items in column ② that you previously indicated using a scale of 1 to 5, one being the least powerful, and five being the most powerful in preventing you from changing the intensity and type of containment at the right time. You may want to add additional qualities about yourself that will interfere with changing your commitment over time in the blank spaces below.

①　✓	②　Rank 1 – 5	③　Containment Change	④　Event, repeated event, personality characteristic, or feeling
			Things that might make you change containment *too early*
			Underestimating how difficult it is for you to attain goals
			A tendency to over-rely on what you feel is correct at a given moment in time
			General resistance to following rules
			Boredom that arises when you practice the same recovery skill over and over
			General dislike for following rules
			Things that might make wait *too long* before changing containment
			Fear of asking for what you need
			A general sense that people do not listen to you
			Fear of change

① ✓	② Rank 1 – 5	③ Containment Change	④ Event, repeated event, personality characteristic, or feeling
			A tendency to repeat behaviors over and over

Domain A: Progress Assessment Form

Containment Review—RecoveryMind Training

This evaluation is completed by both the patient or client (self-assessment) and his or her therapist or staff members. After starting work on a skill, place the approximate start date in the column provided. The patient or client fills out the form first. A therapist or staff member performs the same evaluation, placing a check mark in each row that indicates progress in assigned Recovery Skills. This process may need to be repeated several times as work progresses in each domain.

A check mark in the B column signifies that work has begun. The I column should be checked if the patient is in an intermediate or midway through his or her work on this item, and the C column should be checked if the patient has made sufficient progress in the skill to move forward to his or her next task. Review and discussion of this form helps patients and therapists set clear treatment expectations and recovery goals.

Domain A Recovery Skill	Date: Patient			Staff			Date: Patient			Staff			Date: Patient			Staff		
	B	I	C	B	I	C	B	I	C	B	I	C	B	I	C	B	I	C
Understands basic concepts and types of containment.																		
Intellectually accepts containment as a tool to promote abstinence.																		
Recognizes and has experienced how AddictBrain has altered past thoughts and behaviors.																		
Has identified and practiced current and potential future ways AddictBrain can sabotage recovery.																		
Has a workable plan for addiction containment as treatment intensity decreases.																		
Recognizes how past experiences, emotions, and personality issues may affect containment.																		
Effectively using and modifying containment tools to prevent past experiences, emotions, and personality from sabotaging recovery.																		
Has a workable plan for addiction containment when formal treatment is complete.																		

Domain A: Containment Notes

1.   J. B. Rotter. "Some Problems and Misconceptions Related to the Construct of Internal Versus External Control of Reinforcement." *J Consult Clin Psychol* 43, no. 1 (1975): 56–67.

2.   If you want to refresh your memory as to why this appears to be so, review the earlier chapters of the RecoveryMind Training text.

3.   R. L. DuPont, and G. E. Skipper. "Six Lessons from State Physician Health Programs to Promote Long-Term Recovery." *J Psychoactive Drugs* 44, no. 1 (2012): 72–78.

4.   R. L. DuPont, and G. E. Skipper. "Physician Health Programs - a Model of Successful Treatment of Addiction." *Counselor* Dec (2010): 22–29.

5.   R. DuPont, A. McLellan, W. White, L. Merlo, and M. Gold. "Setting the Standard for Recovery: Physicians' Health Programs." *J Subst Abuse Treat* 36, no. 2 (2009): 159–71.

6.   N. M. Petry. *Contingency Management for Substance Abuse Treatment : A Guide to Implementing This Evidence-Based Practice.* New York: Routledge, 2012.

7.   N. M. Petry, J. Tedford, M. Austin, C. Nich, K. M. Carroll, and B. J. Rounsaville. "Prize Reinforcement Contingency Management for Treating Cocaine Users: How Low Can We Go, and with Whom?". *Addiction* 99, no. 3 (2004): 349–60.

8.   M. Stitzer, and N. Petry. "Contingency Management for Treatment of Substance Abuse." *Annu. Rev. Clin. Psychol.* 2 (2006): 411–34.

9.   One of the greatest educators in our field, Herbert Kleber, M.D., told me many years ago, "Craving is perceived availability." This apothegm has stuck with me ever since.

Domain B: Recovery Basics
Skills Groups, Assignments, Worksheets, and Progress Assessment Form

Chapter Overview

Most clients who have entered treatment or outpatient care begin their journey in Domain A. However, clients should not start in Domain A and just plod sequentially through each of the elements of every RMT domain. Rather, a therapist who implements RecoveryMind Training correctly will consider each client's situation and carefully adjust assignments, group work, and other exercises, tailoring each component to meet that individual's needs. This addresses the valid complaint about addiction treatment today that it is not sufficiently individualized. RecoveryMind Training is highly customizable, responding to that concern. It is also a comprehensive treatment process that provides addiction recovery skills to a wide variety of patients at many levels of care.

Consider a patient who has never been in treatment before, has a low level of psychiatric comorbidity, and enters an intensive outpatient program. If she stays for four weeks or less, you would only expect her to acquire the skills in Domains A and B. In such a case, this may be sufficient to start her recovery journey.

Treatment programs with longer and/or more intense care have sufficient patient contact hours to expand work into the remaining four domains. An individual in this higher intensity care with an extremely hostile self-concept, for example, will need to work in Domain D, and so on.

Work in Domain B is intended for clients who do not know how to use recovery tools. Domain B teaches patients recovery skills in three areas:
1. How to successfully use twelve-step and similar mutual-help programs
2. Learning basic mindfulness techniques
3. Gaining self-insight through the Recovery Reflection

The skills in Domain B help clients schedule recovery activities, develop a daily agenda that promotes their recovery plan, look at past dishonesties, and begin work with the Twelve Steps. A patient then moves on to take stock of how addiction reshaped his or her life and in doing so differentiates him- or herself from his or her addiction disorder. Each of the early exercises prepares the patient for the longest and most difficult assignment in this domain, the addiction life history.

Human beings love stories. We read novels, watch movies, and tell anecdotes about ourselves and about our families, friends, and heroes. Such stories define who we are. Unbeknownst to its hapless victim, AddictBrain has conjured stories in its victims. At first unconsciously and, after a time, consciously, the individual with a substance use disorder identifies with that story. At this point, someone with a substance use disorder accepts these self-deprecating stories as true; the individual is the addiction illness. In Domain B, we drag that story onto paper, so the individual with a substance use disorder can recognize who he or she has become. This opens the door to considering another plot for his or her life—the recovery story. This new story will be expanded by work in Domains C through F and in his or her work in support groups and ongoing psychotherapy.

It is important to understand that we do not *replace* the AddictBrain story with the recovery story. The memories created by AddictBrain are lodged deep within the mind; it would be naïve to think we can kick them aside. Instead, we clarify and acknowledge the patient's understanding of his or her past and in doing so open the door to a new way of living life, to a new story. Both stories remain side by side, the AddictBrain slowly decreasing in intensity over time, replaced by the thoughts, actions, and memories of RecoveryMind.

There are five Skills Groups in Domain B:

B1) Learning how to use the Recovery Reflection to plan daily activities
B2) Mindfulness meditation
B3) Twelve-step concepts
B4) What to expect from twelve-step meetings
B5) How to participate in twelve-step meetings

There are four Assignment Group tasks in Domain B:

B1) Read the *Three by Five* worksheet aloud and receive feedback.
B2) Read the *Honesty, Self-Disclosure, and Asking for Help* worksheet aloud in group therapy and receive feedback.
B3) Read the *What and When* worksheet aloud in Assignment Group. The group provides feedback, including the most honest responses and responses that were minimizing, displacing blame, and lacking in depth.
B4) Read the *Addiction Life History* to the group and ask for feedback. Note that this history is written or typed in free form. I have provided an *Addiction Life History* worksheet, but this simple worksheet only contains instructions and preliminary questions that help focus the longer, freestyle narrative.

There are eight worksheets in Domain B:

B1) The **Recovery Reflection Worksheet**. Patients complete this worksheet daily through the course of treatment. It forms the basis for the methodical self-examination necessary for recovery.

B2) The **Three by Five Worksheet**. This brief exercise is designed to nudge the patient into reevaluating his or her distorted thinking. It is a gentle introduction to self-disclosure and listening to peer feedback.

B3) The **Honesty, Self-Disclosure, and Asking for Help Worksheet**. This worksheet prepares the patient for the important tasks of recovery. It teaches the patient to practice honesty with a difficult subject and disclosure of one or more past or present secrets. The patient reveals these secrets in Assignment Group. The patient then asks another patient for help with a particular issue. Practicing this in Treatment Group prepares them to continue this practice

B4) The **Basics of the Twelve Steps Worksheet**. For patients who are unfamiliar with the twelve-step process or need a refresher, staff can assign this worksheet. It helps patients understand the basics of how to use support groups, how to read and understand the literature, and how to use each step.

B5) The **Twelve Steps Reading Worksheet**. Most patients will benefit from reading assigned chapters in the recovery literature. There are six assignments, to be completed one per week. At the end of each week, each patient hands in his or her worksheet as he or she completes weekly reading assignments. Staff members read each worksheet to confirm there is a growing understanding as well as to learn the patient's reactions to assignments. This worksheet also gently tasks a patient to complete the reading.

B6) The **What and When Worksheet**. This worksheet examines the basic manifestations of addiction, asking the client to examine each. Then the client places each of the different ways his or her addiction expressed itself over time. It examines addiction switching, combining, and other aspects of addiction interaction disorder.[1]

B7) The **Addiction Life History Worksheet**. This worksheet contains instructions and preliminary questions that teach a patient how to write his or her history. A client will use this instructional sheet to improve the depth and content of his or her life history assignment.

B8) The **First Step Summary Worksheet**. This worksheet is the culmination of the patient's work with the first of twelve AA steps. After completing all other items in Domain B, receiving group feedback and revising work as requested by peers and staff, the client completes the First Step worksheet. I think that placing this worksheet last in the list of tasks results in a more thorough and honest First Step.

Domain B: Skills Groups

Skills Group B1: Recovery Reflection

Recovery Reflection creates a conscious, planned way of redirecting one's life. At first it should be conscientiously applied, spending time on the worksheet three times per day. As the client progresses, the reflection process is slowly internalized and the actual pen to paper activities decrease. Once learned, the client and his therapist drop the mid-day element (⊙) first, often after two to three weeks. The morning element is dropped much later; it helps the client organize the day, preventing AddictBrain from sneaking into his daily activities. Many clients continue the evening Recovery Reflection for years on a more abbreviated form.

Table B.1: Recovery Reflection

Element	Description	Time of Day	Purpose
1	Recovery Schedule		Important recovery activities must be scheduled each day to prevent spontaneous AddictBrain responses.
2	Mindfulness Meditation		Meditation calms the mind, helping you be less reactive to strong emotions. It decreases craving in most people.
3	Emotional Awareness		Naming and noticing feeling states prevents the person in recovery from unconscious acting out emotions.
4	Deception Detection		Patients catalog dishonesties to self and others. This element breaks the internal and external lies that AddictBrain uses to hide.
5	Craving Recognition		Patients record recent cravings and their relationship to events, thoughts, and feelings. This will build a relapse prevention plan.
6	Healthy Attachment		Patients must learn healthy attachments to recover. This element looks at connection styles and problems.
7	Step Review		Each day the patient records work on the Twelve Steps, tracking any change in her understanding and attitude about the recovery process.
8	Issue Identification		Here the patient builds a list of emotional and interpersonal issues that need attention over the next several days.

The Recovery Reflection skill is best trained over two or more sessions. In the first session, the daily reflection is introduced. The leader hands out a Recovery Reflection worksheet (at the end of this chapter) to each member. The leader then describes the first element of Recovery Reflection and has patients complete this one section. Group feedback then ensues. Through the process of group sharing, new members learn how to execute each element within the Recovery Reflection. Group members who have been through this training describe how it has helped them keep a focus on recovery. The group leader describes how Recovery Reflection continues through recovery. Two to three of the elements should be described, discussed, and practiced in each Skills Group. A separate Skills Group teaches mindfulness meditation. A patient will begin new parts of the Recovery Reflection when he or she has completed training in the corresponding Skills Groups. For clients in individual therapy, the therapist teaches them how to use the worksheet.

Several pragmatic points need to be taught regarding the Recovery Reflection. Patients are instructed to turn in the previous day's Recovery Reflection to staff each morning if they are in milieu-based treatment (ASAM Levels 2 through 4). In individual treatment (commonly, ASAM Level 1) the therapist works with the client to decide how to handle form submission. Early on, a therapist might request the client fax the form daily at first. Later, the client might bring the week's Recovery Reflections to be briefly reviewed at the start of each session. The contents of the Recovery Reflection may or may not be part of the patient or client's record. These forms establish daily self-care and track treatment progress.

Skills Group B2: Mindfulness Meditation

An expanding body of knowledge supports the use of mindfulness meditation in addiction recovery.[2–6] Mindfulness meditation has proved especially effective in relapse prevention.[6,4] Mindfulness meditation is not in and of itself a religious practice. Caregivers may need to reassert this point several times with clients who live by a strong religious doctrine or who are opposed to religion or atheist.

Mindfulness meditation encourages contemplation, discourages impulsive action, increases a patient's tolerance of distressing emotions, and increases his or her sense of connectedness and spirituality. In a single individual session or Skills Group, the leader introduces the topic of mindfulness meditation. The leader explains the benefits of mindfulness meditation. A brief question-and-answer period then ensues where patients discuss their previous experiences with meditation. A common response from addicted individuals (who are used to dramatic effects from alcohol or other drugs or addictive behaviors) is "I tried it, and it didn't do much." The leader gently points out that meditation must be practiced for some time to be effective; the benefits are cumulative and realized slowly. Next, the leader encourages everyone to attempt a brief episode of mindfulness meditation. The patients sit upright in chairs during initial training. The room should be sound-shielded to prevent extraneous noise from interrupting the experience. As a patient becomes more comfortable, he or she should consider other modifications such as sitting on the floor on a mat, meditating outside, and so forth. Different leaders may teach this in a different manner;[7–9] however, the basic steps include:

1. Sit in a comfortable physical posture, either
   a. On a mat with a straight but not rigid back; or
   b. Upright in a chair, avoid resting against the back if this is comfortable.
2. Remove unnecessary objects from your lap and your immediate area. Remove a ticking watch or uncomfortable eyeglasses.
3. Scan the body and relax as much possible. Place your hands on your thighs or rest them gently in your lap.
4. You may choose to allow your face to relax into a half smile. Your mouth may fall open just a bit.
5. Allow the eyes to gently close and turn the mind inward.
6. Begin focusing on the breath as it causes the chest to rise and fall. An alternative is to notice the air as it enters and exits through the nose or to follow your abdomen as it distends and retracts with each breath.
7. If distracted by thought, either label the thought as "thinking" or watch the thought drift away as if it is carried on a leaf down a stream.
8. If distracted for a several seconds, gently return to focusing on the breath. Avoid judgment about distractions.
9. Avoid abrupt movements. If possible, avoid any movement with the exception of movements created by the breath.
10. When it is time to stop, keep the eyes closed for a moment while your thoughts return to the room.
11. Slowly open the eyes, looking at a neutral object. Slowly return to your surroundings and sit still for a moment.

The leader should start with brief one to two-minute meditation sessions, followed by group (or individual) discussion of the experience. Through the discussion, the leader reinforces the important principles of meditation including compassion to self, recognition of the chatter in one's mind, letting that chatter go, and returning the focus to the breath. Some patients will be unable to meditate in any meaningful way. Such patients might be directed to supervised meditation or sound technology that induces meditative states.[10]

Skills Group B3: Twelve-Step Concepts

The first task in this group is introducing the basic twelve-step literature. Using a discussion format, several core twelve-step books are introduced to group members. The leader should bring several copies of each book to the session. While discussing a book, copies are passed around the room. The leader describes the difference between core literature (used in treatment) and ancillary books (Chuck C's *A New Pair of Glasses*, Ernie Kurtz's *Not God*, and others.). Core literature is the first thing patients should read in treatment. Brief discussions about the following texts should occur, describing the treatment-based reading assignments in each:

- *Alcoholics Anonymous: Fourth Edition* (The AA Big Book)
- *The Twelve Steps and Twelve Traditions* (The AA Twelve and Twelve)
- *Narcotics Anonymous 6th Edition* (The NA Basic Text)

Remember to emphasize that much of the literature, especially the AA Big Book, was written quite some time ago. The style may seem outdated or awkward to our twenty-first century ears. However, the principles hold true. Patients may find themselves rebelling against concepts in the twelve-step literature. When this occurs staff should become curious (i.e., "What part did you have the most trouble with? Why do you think this is the case?"), rather than directive (i.e., "You should go back and try to read that chapter with an open mind."). I have learned over the years that AA readings are like a Rorschach ink blot: they reflect on the unconscious constructs of the addicted mind, often providing windows into past abuse, difficulties with religion or authority figures, and so forth.

The second task is introducing the steps. Many patients will come to treatment with preconceived notions about the steps or with varying levels of understanding. If this education is in a group, encourage participants to teach each other. Emphasize that, when it comes to the steps, a slower and more thorough approach is best.

Hand out and discuss Table B2. Encourage members to describe examples of the character problems that exist and how each step will help them overcome them with involved with the principal and action involved with each step.

Table B2: Principles behind the First Five Steps

Step		Character Problem	Principle	Action
1	We admitted we were powerless over alcohol (addiction)—that our lives had become unmanageable.	Deception and Dishonesty	Honesty	Surrender
2	Came to believe that a Power greater than ourselves could restore us to sanity.	Self-will and Disbelief	Hope	Realization
3	Made a decision to turn our will and our lives over to the care of God, as we understood Him.	Self-will and Fear	Faith	Ask for and accept help
4	Made a searching and fearless moral inventory of ourselves.	Self-pity and Isolation	Courage	Self-examination
5	Admitted to God, to ourselves, and to another human being the exact nature of our wrongs.	False Pride	Integrity	Open Communication

The third task is introducing reading assignments. All patients should read parts of the basic literature before they leave treatment. Too often, this is left to chance. We ensure that patients read and consider what they have read by writing their thoughts down on Worksheet B5. Here are the reading assignments, in an approximate reading order:

1. AA Big Book:[11] Chapter 1
2. AA Big Book: Chapter 2
3. AA Big Book: The Doctor's Opinion
4. AA Big Book: Chapter 5
5. AA Twelve and Twelve[12]: Chapter 1

The individual therapist assigns the readings to his or her client or, if in organized treatment, patients may discuss how best to complete reading and form completion in a group setting. Patients are instructed to return Worksheet B5 for review once it is complete.

Skills Group B4: What Are Twelve-Step Meetings?

Patients will arrive in treatment with a wide variety of previous experiences with support groups such as Alcoholics Anonymous. Research has shown that patients respond to AA and its sister organizations in many ways. Some individuals find deep connections and meeting in twelve-step groups. Others find them helpful but not deeply rewarding. A third group struggles mightily with support groups. Part of this response comes from inadequate preparation and a lack of understanding of what these groups do.

The best way to get the largest percentage of patients to use the inexpensive and often invaluable help of twelve-step meetings is education followed by sufficient exposure. This Skills Group teaches patients how to use twelve-step meetings to sustain recovery. Unfortunately, this Skills Group cannot be reproduced in individual therapy. It combines teaching, discussion, and role-playing. Feel free to role-play any part of this Skills Group; doing so will increase meaningful retention.

In this group, the therapist has four tasks. He or she will
1. Describe how twelve-step meetings are run
2. Discuss what meetings do
3. Increase understanding of what occurs in meetings
4. Provide practice in getting comfortable in meetings

The leader begins Skills Group B4 with a *short* description of the history of Alcoholics Anonymous. One helpful approach is to start with "Addiction is a complex, pervasive disease. We must use all resources at our fingertips to fight it. Some of you will embrace twelve-step recovery, some will find meetings helpful, and some may feel resistant to them or find them less helpful."

It is imperative that this presentation be limited to five minutes or less. The leader then describes the many variants of AA and who they are designed for. Depending on the composition of patients, the leader may discuss AA, NA, CA, CMA, AlAnon, GA, SA, SAA, OA, DA, CODA, and ACA and others. It is important to describe the subtle differences in meetings and the different manifestations of addiction that each meeting type addresses.

To segue to the next task, I suggest the leader ask the question: *"What do meetings do to help with recovery?"* Then through the course of the discussion, the leader hopes to hear many or all the effects noted in the list below. Feel free to add you own effects to this list.

Twelve-Step meetings:
- Create a social network of individuals who do not use alcohol and/or other drugs and are focused on recovery
- Improve interpersonal skills
- Build self-acceptance through the sharing of common stories
- Correct thought and feeling distortions produced by AddictBrain
- Provide a daily reminder of the importance of keeping recovery as a central focus
- Generate a sense of belonging

- Decrease addiction-induced shame
- Provide opportunities to study the literature
- Provide practical skills to prevent relapse
- Normalize the disturbing experience of craving, euphoric recall, self-destructive patterns, and so forth, and places the blame for them on the illness and not on the individual
- Encourage personal responsibility for recovery
- Create a roadmap to a different way of living that increases the probability of sobriety/abstinence

As an item is brought up, the leader asks the group members for an example or vignette that describes this effect. Allow discussion to continue if group members develop insight or find relief in any particular item.

The leader describes the types of meetings. Discussion meetings, speaker's meetings, step meetings, Big Book meetings, and traditions meetings are described. The reasons one goes to each of these meeting types is important.

Because discussion meetings are the most common, the leader describes its components, stopping after each component for group interaction. A suggested list of components to explain includes:

1. The introductory reading. The introductory reading is designed to focus all attendees on the purpose of the meeting and to reinforce the basic principles of change inherent in the twelve-step process.
2. If the meeting is a discussion meeting, a topic is called from participants. Because AA is leaderless, feedback is discouraged. This helps all attendees focus on the principle discussed and prevents comments that are hurtful to the participants.
3. In a discussion meeting, individual provide different types of wisdom. These include, but are not limited to:
   a. Gratitude for how one's life is today
   b. Specific suggestions about relapse prevention techniques
   c. Insights learned along the spiritual journey of recovery
   d. Discussion of a personal experience that demonstrates how to implement a specific recovery principle
   e. Sharing of a common pitfall or problem. This normalizes some of the painful or difficult aspects of life.
   f. Teaching other members to "not do what I did."
   g. Unburdening a member's anguish

Different meetings conclude in different ways. Many celebrate time in recovery through a token contingency management system. In AA, this is called the "chip system." This may be followed by a group prayer.

When patients begin attending meetings, you should ask patients what they heard, felt, and reacted to, gently coaxing them is the most effective manner of using this invaluable resource. If a client launches into his or her dislike of meetings, the therapist should use supportive listening. Avoid lectures about how AA and NA have saved thousands of lives and such. Each patient will go on to use meetings and the twelve-step system in his or her own way or not at all.

One wise psychiatrist said, "Of course people with substance use disorders do not like meetings—that is the very problem!" When open-minded individuals who do not have an addiction disorder attend their first AA meeting, the most common response when leaving is "That was a wonderful experience! Everyone should have a support network like that!" A person's personality, twisted by AddictBrain, has an inherent dislike of AA meetings because they threaten the chaos of addiction that ensures continued use and chaos caused by the disease. That said, even when AddictBrain's influence is lessened, there are those who remain unable to get anything out of AA. The therapist helps his or her client search out additional support from other sources in such cases.

Skills Group B5: Attending Twelve-Step Meetings

The only task in this Skills Group is helping patients achieve a modicum of comfort in recovery support groups. Like Skills Group B3 above, it cannot be reproduced in individual therapy. However, the individual therapist can and should review a client's response to meetings *in situ*, searching for ways of finding value and comfort with this important recovery tool. I have found over the years that overcoming internal resistance to attending meetings is one of the most important tasks of treatment.

The leader starts this group emphasizing the importance of becoming comfortable in meetings. This is especially true for patients with social phobia. The leader directs the bulk of members to sit in a circle as if they are waiting for a meeting. Empty chairs are scattered through the circle, especially in the chairs farthest from the door. Several members are sent outside, and when signaled, they enter the room, scan for a seat, and discuss their anxiety or discomfort. Some principles to role-play are:
- Sit where you feel safe.
- When you become comfortable, introduce yourself to at least one new person each meeting.
- Come early and listen to conversations that are recovery related.
- Stay afterward, standing next to someone who shared in a meaningful way.

- Avoid congregating in groups with other patients from your facility.
- You may sit with one person from treatment but find a place to sit next to someone else on your other side.
- Listen for the message that is coming through beneath the stores that are told. *Hear the meta-message.*
- Ask how a topic applies to you as often as you tell yourself you cannot relate to something being said.

Make sure members with anxiety or resistance have practiced entering and settling in the room. When this is complete, recreate a mock snippet of an AA meeting. What makes this snippet different, however, is the leader stops and starts this meeting frequently (every two or three minutes) to encourage discussion by the members of the Skills Group. The leader microdissects comments of those who are sitting within the meeting, restructuring their experience and teaching them how to use what is shared to build recovery. Group members are encouraged to vocalize positive and negative feelings about what has been discussed. Such work trains members to effectively listen and process meeting content.

This Skills Group may span one or more sessions to help its members get the most out of support group attendance.

Domain B: Assignment Group Tasks

Assignment Group Task B1: The Three by Five

The Three by Five is commonly one of a patient or client's first assignments. The purpose of the Three by Five is to acclimate patients to presenting assignments in group therapy and receiving group feedback. There is no need to assign it to patients who are comfortable with group therapy and self-disclosure nor to patients who have accepted they have an illness. It is a simple exercise that asks patients to begin the process of critically examining their illness. If assigned, the patient should complete it within a few days or before the next individual appointment.

Using the appropriate worksheet, the patient lists five triggers for use, five high-risk situations, and five life consequences produced by his or her addiction. He or she then reads the worksheet in Assignment Group. Other members of the group provide feedback about the honesty, directness, and depth of disclosure. Should a patient fail to complete the assignment in a thorough fashion, the leader collects the feedback and gently directs the patient to revise the assignment prior to a second presentation. The therapist may need to structure feedback from time to time to prevent members from unconsciously expressing their own hostile introjects onto others.

Assignment Group Task B2: Honesty, Self-Disclosure, and Asking for Help

This Assignment Group task teaches patients three important recovery skills. AddictBrain drives the addicted individual to dishonesty, to withhold information from others, and to dismiss or devalue the support and feedback that comes from friends and loved ones. This group is somewhat different from other Assignment Groups in that the accompanying worksheet is filled out in the actual session. As many group members as possible share their responses with the group.

The group is divided into three components, one for each part of the assignment. During the first component, each participant writes down one past dishonesty or deceit. Taking turns, each member reads the dishonesty to the group and follows this with the truth. The leader structures the group, reinforcing deeper confessions when possible.

The group then turns to self-disclosure. Each member writes down something from his or her past that he or she has withheld from friends or loved ones. Then, going around the room, each participant discloses this information to others in the group. A variant is to place the slips of paper in a pile and have members pick up each other's statements. More intense self-disclosure is rewarded by group acknowledgment.

Finally, each member of the group writes down a request for help. These often emerge out of the first two group issues. That is, a participant might ask for help being more honest about a past secret to others or ask for support when self-disclosing something to family. The group ends with a reiteration of the importance of confidentiality and not discussing the contents of this group outside of the room.

This task may wind up requiring more than one session. Remember, this group can be scary and painful. The extra practice should be accommodated if time is available. The leader may urge a patient to also continue discussion of a topic in Process Group.

Assignment Group Task B3: The What and When

During this group, the assigned patient reads the contents of her completed Worksheet B6, the What and When Worksheet. As in all similar assignments, the protagonist reads a section and asks for feedback. Other members ask questions, working as a team to uncover self-deception and to dislodge resistance to self-acceptance. Non-protagonist members are encouraged to share their own similar experiences (e.g., "*I drove my young children in the car after smoking pot, never thinking I was putting them in danger.*"). However, non-protagonist members should be prevented from diverting the focus on the work of the current protagonist. (This, by the way, is one of the main differences from Process Group).

Assignment Group Task B4: Reading Your Addiction Life History

After a patient completes and submits Worksheet B7: Addiction Life History, his or her therapist reviews the written narrative for completeness. Often the case manager may request revisions of some parts of this complex assignment.

As soon as the patient completes any needed revisions, the case manager assigns a date when the patient will read his or her Addiction Life History in Assignment Group. When completing this assignment in group, the patient does not methodically read the items on the B7 worksheet; rather, the purpose of this worksheet is only to structure and deepen the patient's subsequent Addiction Life History.

Before the life history is read, the leader instructs members of the group to listen and reflect on elements of the history that are like their own. The leader structures the group members to be respectful and attentive. Patients are urged to consider themes rather than details. If they hear the protagonist describe a consequence of his or her disease, they can ask themselves "Has this happened to me?" and, if not

"Could this happen to me in the future?" Group participants are also asked to note minimizations and rationalizations that the protagonist describes in his or her story. Participants should also make note of blame, projection, entitlement, and other defenses that appear in the story. When these difficulties are pointed out to the protagonist during feedback at the end, the individual who points out a defense *must* describe the manner in which he or she uses the defense. By reading the addiction life history each member is encouraged to increase her or his self-insight.

More than any other assignment, presenting the Addiction Life History should be painfully honest and direct. In the group, the protagonist is subject to primitive misinterpretations of minor slights. He or she may misperceive constructive or supportive feedback as derisive or attacking.

The history is read through in its entirety. Only the briefest interruptions are allowed, usually to clarify a timeframe, word, or concept. No one may enter or leave group during the reading or comment period.

Once the history has been read and other group members provide feedback, the group works as a team to help the protagonist complete the Worksheet B8: First Step Summary. The group may want the protagonist to think about this worksheet and read it aloud the next time the Assignment Group convenes.

Domain B: Recovery Basics Worksheets

Overview of Worksheets

This domain teaches patients the basic skills needed for recovery. You will find that some of the skills introduced in Domain B are expanded upon in subsequent Domains C through F. This is intentional and partly comes from the fact that twelve-step programs promote emotional resiliency (Domain C), restructure a patient's internal narrative (Domain D), are based upon spirituality (Domain E), and teach relapse prevention (Domain F). In many ways, RecoveryMind Training expands the scope and makes explicit the subtler aspects of twelve-step recovery.

For those patients without significant comorbid conditions (depression, personality problems, past trauma, pain disorders, or other physical or mental challenges) treatment may be limited to Domains A and B. Patients with more extensive needs require more extensive and nuanced treatment. This occurs in Domains C though F.

When working in Domain B, a center must have ready access to a library of related literature. Some patients may respond to reading Alcoholics Anonymous literature, while others may need to be assigned reading in derivative literature.

Eight worksheets are available for Domain B. In patients who need work in this area, the worksheets should be accomplished in order and at a pace dictated by patient readiness and the intensity of the treatment system (commonly these are accomplished more rapidly in an ASAM Level 3.5 or 2.5 program than in an outpatient therapist's office).

B1) The **Recovery Reflection** Worksheet refocuses patients on the daily tasks of recovery.

B2) The **Three by Five** Worksheet starts the discovery process about problems caused by substance use.

B3) The **Honesty** Worksheet explores how AddictBrain hides through dishonesty.

B4) The **Basics of the Twelve Steps** Worksheet introduces the patient to twelve-step recovery.

B5) The **Twelve-Step Reading** Worksheet structures early reading and reading reflection about twelve-step literature.

B6) The **What and When** Worksheet builds an addiction timeline.

B7) The **Addiction History** Worksheet deepens a patient's understanding related to the progression of his or her illness.

B8) The **First-Step Summary** Worksheet prepares a patient to work the first of the Twelve Steps with a temporary sponsor or staff. Patients in extended care treatment will complete additional worksheets for Steps Two through Five, depending on the time available.

Worksheet B1: Recovery Reflection

Morning Reflection

Name: _____ Date: _____ Time in Recovery: _____

Recovery Schedule

My first goal is to remain sober and to continue to grow in recovery. Today I will:

1) Attend a twelve-step meeting at this time _____ and this location _____

2) Focus my attention on this step _____ in this manner (read, write discuss a particular feeling or thought) _____

3) Spend time on the phone, in electronic communication, or in person with _____.

   I will ask them for help with _____

   _____

4) I have this specific issue I want to discuss with others in recovery today _____

   _____

5) This particular emotion is especially important for me to experience / avoid / explore / feel / talk about _____

6) I have made a commitment to myself or others to accomplish these additional tasks:

   a) _____

   b) _____

   c) _____

   d) _____

Mindfulness Meditation

The next task in your reflection is Mindfulness Meditation. Find a quiet place and sit upright in a chair, your hands resting softly on your thighs. You may choose to place your hands in positions that you have learned in meditation skills training. Allow your eyes to close gently. Relax your face with just a hint of a smile. Focus on your breath as it moves in and out of your nose or mouth. When a thought, urge, or feeling comes to you, watch it drift away like a leaf going down a stream. If you become distracted, gently return to your breath. Practice this at first for several minutes and extend this time as you become more comfortable. When the meditation time is up, slowly open your eyes and sit for a moment, reacquainting yourself with your surroundings. If you are unable to meditate, you may use one of the audio files that help with mindfulness. You will learn more about meditation and its recovery benefits during your time with us in treatment.

Emotional Awareness

In the time since your last Recovery Reflection, you may have experienced strong or surprising feelings or emotions. This is normal in treatment and recovery. Record these feelings below. Place an asterisk after any feeling that was especially uncomfortable or one you wanted to suppress or avoid.

Since my last Recovery Reflection, I noticed the following feelings or emotions:

_____ , related to _____

_____ , related to _____

_____ , related to _____

_____ , related to _____

Deception Detection

Addiction produces some level of dishonesty in every one of its victims. Please write about any deceptions, dishonesties, or lies you have thought or uttered to another person since your last reflection. Do not ignore seemingly small dishonesties or "white lies" here either. Dig deep for the lies you have told repeatedly or long ago. Place an asterisk next to any of these you need to disclose and discuss in group therapy (even if you are not ready yet to do so). Fill out the blanks below, describing the deception or dishonesty in full. Then check *each* box (☑) below that describes the type of dishonesty.

Deception or Dishonesty: _____

_____

This occurred in the: ☐ Past several days   ☐ Recent past   ☐ In my past   ☐ Is it ongoing?

This deception is: ☐ Shading the truth   ☐ Self-deception   ☐ Dishonest to others
           ☐ Related to my addiction

Deception or Dishonesty: _____

_____

This occurred in the: ☐ Past several days   ☐ Recent past   ☐ Distant past   ☐ Is it ongoing?

This deception is: ☐ Shading the truth   ☐ Self-deception   ☐ Lied to others
           ☐ Related to my addiction

Deception or Dishonesty: _____

_____

This occurred in the: ☐ Past several days   ☐ Recent past   ☐ Distant past   ☐ Is it ongoing?

This deception is: ☐ Shading the truth   ☐ Self-deception   ☐ Lied to others
           ☐ Related to my addiction

Craving Recognition

Describe and rate craving events you have experienced since your last Recovery Reflection. If you have not been trained in using the RecoveryMind craving scale, skip the check boxes. If you have, fill out the check boxes below.

Craving Description: _____

_____

_____

Intensity rating: ☐ One   ☐ Two   ☐ Three   ☐ Four   ☐ Five

The craving: ☐ Is a conditioned trigger, from this trigger _____

                ☐ Is emotions-based, from the feeling _____

                ☐ Is memory-induced, from the memory of _____

Craving Description: _____

_____

_____

Intensity rating: ☐ One   ☐ Two   ☐ Three   ☐ Four   ☐ Five

The craving: ☐ Is a conditioned trigger, from this trigger _____

                ☐ Is emotions-based, from the feeling _____

                ☐ Is memory-induced, from the memory of _____

☀ *Midday Reflection*

Name: _____ Date _____

Mindfulness Meditation

Spend five to fifteen minutes in mindfulness meditation. Meditation slows down your thinking and allows you to contemplate your day and find peace in emotional turmoil.

Emotional Awareness

In the time since your last Recovery Reflection, you may have experienced strong or surprising feelings or emotions. This is normal in treatment and recovery. Record these feelings below. Place an asterisk after any feeling that was especially uncomfortable or one you wanted to suppress or avoid.

Since my last Recovery Reflection, I noticed the following feelings or emotions:

_____ , related to _____

_____ , related to _____

_____ , related to _____

_____ , related to _____

Deception Detection

Write about any deceptions, dishonesties, or lies you have thought or uttered to another person since your last reflection. Do not ignore seemingly small dishonesties or "white lies." Enter them here as well. Dig deep for the lies you told long ago or repeatedly. Place an asterisk next to any of these you need to disclose and discuss in group therapy (even if you are not ready yet to do so). Fill out the blanks below, describing the deception or dishonesty in full. Then check *each* box (☑) below that describes the type of dishonesty.

Deception or Dishonesty: _____

_____

This occurred in the: ☐ Past several days   ☐ Recent past   ☐ In my past   ☐ Is it ongoing?

This deception is: ☐ Shading the truth   ☐ Self-Deception   ☐ Dishonest to others
                     ☐ Related to my addiction

Deception or Dishonesty: _____

_____

This occurred in the: ☐ Past several days   ☐ Recent past   ☐ Distant past   ☐ Is it ongoing?

This deception is: ☐ Shading the truth   ☐ Self-Deception   ☐ Lied to others
                     ☐ Related to my addiction

Deception or Dishonesty: _____

_____

This occurred in the: ☐ Past several days   ☐ Recent past   ☐ Distant past   ☐ Is it ongoing?

This deception is: ☐ Shading the truth   ☐ Self-Deception   ☐ Lied to others
                     ☐ Related to my addiction

Craving Recognition

Describe and rate craving events you have experienced since your last Recovery Reflection. If you have
not been trained in using the RecoveryMind craving scale, skip the check boxes. If you have, fill out the
check boxes below.

Craving Description: _____

_____

_____

Intensity rating: ☐ One ☐ Two ☐ Three ☐ Four ☐ Five

The craving: ☐ Is a conditioned trigger, from this trigger _____

               ☐ Is emotions-based, from the feeling _____

               ☐ Is memory-induced, from the memory of _____

Craving Description: _____

_____

_____

Intensity rating: ☐ One ☐ Two ☐ Three ☐ Four ☐ Five

The craving: ☐ Is a conditioned trigger, from this trigger _____

               ☐ Is emotions-based, from the feeling _____

               ☐ Is memory-induced, from the memory of _____

🌙 *Evening Reflection*

Name: _____ Date _____

Mindfulness Meditation

Spend five to fifteen minutes in mindfulness meditation. Meditation slows down your thinking and allows you to contemplate your day and find peace in emotional turmoil.

Emotional Awareness

In the time since your last Recovery Reflection, you may have experienced strong or surprising feelings or emotions. This is normal in treatment and recovery. Record these feelings below. Place an asterisk after any feeling that was especially uncomfortable or one you wanted to suppress or avoid.

Since my last Recovery Reflection, I noticed the following feelings or emotions:

_____ , related to _____

_____ , related to _____

_____ , related to _____

_____ , related to _____

Deception Detection

Write about any deceptions, dishonesties, or lies you have thought or uttered to another person since your last reflection. Do not ignore seemingly small dishonesties or "white lies," enter them here as well. Dig deep for dishonesties you told long ago or repeatedly. Place an asterisk next to any of these you need to disclose and discuss in group therapy (even if you are not ready yet to do so). Fill out the blanks below, describing the deception or dishonesty in full. Then check *each* box (☑) below that describes the type of dishonesty.

Deception or Dishonesty: _____

_____

This occurred in the: ☐ Past several days ☐ Recent past ☐ In my past ☐ Is it ongoing?

This deception is: ☐ Shading the truth ☐ Self-Deception ☐ Dishonest to others
☐ Related to my addiction

Deception or Dishonesty: _____

_____

This occurred in the: ☐ Past several days ☐ Recent past ☐ Distant past ☐ Is it ongoing?

This deception is: ☐ Shading the truth ☐ Self-Deception ☐ Lied to others
☐ Related to my addiction

Deception or Dishonesty: _____

_____

This occurred in the: ☐ Past several days ☐ Recent past ☐ Distant past ☐ Is it ongoing?

This deception is: ☐ Shading the truth ☐ Self-Deception ☐ Lied to others
☐ Related to my addiction

Craving Recognition

Describe and rate craving events you have experienced since your last Recovery Reflection. If you have not been trained in using the RecoveryMind craving scale, skip the check boxes. If you have, fill out the check boxes below.

Craving Description: _____

_____

_____

Intensity rating: ☐ One   ☐ Two   ☐ Three   ☐ Four   ☐ Five

The craving: ☐ Is a conditioned trigger, from this trigger _____

☐ Is emotions-based, from the feeling _____

☐ Is memory-induced, from the memory of _____

Craving Description: _____

_____

_____

Intensity rating: ☐ One   ☐ Two   ☐ Three   ☐ Four   ☐ Five

The craving: ☐ Is a conditioned trigger, from this trigger _____

☐ Is emotions-based, from the feeling _____

☐ Is memory-induced, from the memory of _____

Healthy Attachment

Human beings need each other to survive. Our natural temperament and our past experiences form the basis of how we connect or attach to other people in our lives and whether the attachment is healthy or unhealthy. AddictBrain exaggerates unhealthy attachment and suppresses healthy connections. In treatment and early recovery, we have to reevaluate our modes of interacting with those around us. Make a note of at least one episode today where you experienced a connection to another person. Describe what was important about the connection. Describe how you felt and the elements of the connection that were healthy and unhealthy. Briefly note ways you plan to make it better in the days ahead.

Describe the connection experience: _____

_____

What feelings did you experience? What was significant about this experience? _____

_____

_____

What was healthy about the interaction? (Examples: I expressed my feelings clearly; I expressed gratitude for the time with them; I was angry without attacking.) _____

_____

_____

What was unhealthy about the interaction? (Examples: I was verbally hurtful; I made fun of them; I was so interested in them that I lost sight of myself.) _____

_____

_____

Step Review

When we "work the steps," we seek understanding of what a step means, notice our reaction to it, and consider how it applies to us. We discuss our reactions to twelve-step concepts with others. We must also write down our work about each step. If we keep our thoughts in our head and do not write them down, the change of recovery does not occur. In the last section of the Recovery Reflection, review your thoughts and reactions. Consider both the positive and the negative. Do not write what you think others want to hear. At the same time, remain open to change.

The step I committed to work on today was Step ____.

What I learned about this step today was _____

_____

I resist or struggle with the parts of this step. They are _____

_____

I find relief or acceptance in what this step teaches. They are _____

_____

I have noticed a change in my attitude or acceptance about this step, in that _____

_____

Worksheet B2: The Three by Five

With this worksheet, we begin a path of discovery about your problems with substance use or behavioral problems. This is the first of several worksheets that help you define the problem and to learn a language to think about and discuss these problems.

Triggers: Spend a moment thinking about your problems with alcohol, other drugs, or your addictive behaviors. Consider things in the environment, people, situations, or emotions that triggered you to use. As you review these triggers, list five important ones below.

1. _____

2. _____

3. _____

4. _____

5. _____

High-Risk Situations: Consider five situations from your past that always seemed to result in alcohol or other drug use or addictive behaviors. These are called *high-risk situations*. Some may be obvious (e.g., going to your favorite sports bar intending to watch the game). Some may not be so obvious. Search for the more intense high-risk situations and write them down below.

1. _____

2. _____

3. _____

4. _____

5. _____

Negative Consequences: Think about some of the negative consequences of your addiction. Try to list consequences that are the most painful or problematic, the ones that make you cringe when you think of them. Write them down here.

1. _____

2. _____

3. _____

4. _____

5. _____

Worksheet B3: Honesty, Self-Disclosure, and Asking for Help

Spend a minute quieting your mind and centering your thoughts. Then scan through events of your past for a painful or embarrassing dishonesty. The dishonesty does not have to be related to your addiction.

Write it down here. _____

_____

_____

Next write down the truth of that situation. _____

_____

_____

_____

Next, write down a secret from your past, preferably one that you have not told another human being. Describe the secret and information surrounding it in several sentences. _____

_____   _____

_____

_____

Lastly, write down something that you need help with. It may be related to the previous dishonesty or secret. You may ask a friend in treatment to help you tell the truth to a family member. Alternatively, you might want to ask someone to help you disclose a secret to someone else. Write down your request here.

_____

_____

_____

Worksheet B4: The Basics of the Twelve Steps

This worksheet helps you remember the basic knowledge you need to begin using twelve-step meetings. Although we will ask you your understanding of the elements of support groups, this is not a test. Rather we will use this form to make sure you have the essential knowledge to use support group attendance to strengthen your recovery.

Each item will first ask you to define or describe a piece of information or a concept. Fill out your answer *without looking it up or consulting someone else.* We will ask if you feel confident in your understanding. If you check "I need to learn more about his concept," then read more about the concept from the reference materials we provide or ask other patients for help. Then, fill out the second blank labeled "updated answer."

If you do not check the box, this means you feel confident in understanding the item or concept and you can go on to the next question. Remember, the purpose of this exercise is learning. There is no grade, and there are not exact answers. This exercise examines your understanding of the basic principles of twelve-step recovery.

Question 1: In your own words, describe the first step. _____

_____

☐ I need to learn more about this. After research, my revised answer appears below.

_____

_____

Question 2: List three books you will use to learn about twelve-step recovery. Briefly describe their purpose. _____

_____

_____

☐ I need to learn more about this. After research, my revised answer appears below.

_____

_____

_____

Question 3: List three ways in which twelve-step meetings might be beneficial to you. _____

_____

_____

☐ I need to learn more about this. After research, my revised answer appears below.

_____

_____

_____

Question 4: List three things that might get in the way of using twelve-step meetings to assist in your recovery. _____

_____

_____

☐ I need to learn more about this. After research, my revised answer appears below.

_____

_____

_____

Worksheet B5: Twelve-Step Reading

This worksheet promotes reflection after each reading assignment in the basic twelve-step recovery literature.

Read each assignment and then spend a few moments thinking about what you have read. Then complete your responses to each question below. Hand in this sheet at the end of each week and begin the next reading assignment. Your case manager will review this worksheet, returning it to you so that you may record your thoughts about the next reading assignment.

Remember there are no right or wrong answers we are looking for. Answer honestly, so we can match treatment to your current needs. It is normal to struggle with some concepts in treatment and recovery. In fact, we would wonder if you did not have challenges. At the same time, give the readings a chance. Think about what you have read and try to apply what you have read to your own life in your answers below.

Reading Assignment 1, AA Big Book, Chapter 1

Question 1: What ideas or events did you relate to in "Bill's Story?" _____

_____

_____

What parts of "Bill's Story" did you *not* relate to, and why? _____

_____

_____

Reading Assignment 2, AA Big Book, Chapter 2

Question 2: Translating the statements about alcohol to your drug or behavior of choice, where do you see yourself on the addiction spectrum? Please answer honcotly.

☐ User   ☐ Problematic user   ☐ Possible addiction illness
☐ Certain addiction illness   ☐ Severe addiction illness

Why do you place yourself in this place on the continuum?

_____

_____

_____

_____

Reading Assignment 3, AA Big Book, "The Doctors Opinion"

Question 3: Medicine has come a long way since 1939. Still the concept of "an allergy of the body" seems helpful in thinking about addiction. Do you relate to this phrase? Why or why not?

_____

_____

Question 4: Dr. Silkworth writes about a "psychic change" that frees the individual with alcoholism from the obsession. What might that look like for you?

_____

_____

_____

Reading Assignment 4, AA Big Book, Chapter 5

Question 5: Think about this sentence: *"Rarely have we seen a person fail who has thoroughly followed our path."*

What are your positive and negative reactions to it? _____

_____

_____

Question 6: Read the Twelve Steps that start on the second page of Chapter 5. What parts of this list of actions strike you negatively or do you have reactions against? _____

_____

What parts of this list of actions strike you positively or are you attracted to? _____

_____

_____

Reading Assignment 5, Twelve Steps and Twelve Traditions, *Step One*

Question 7: Is it difficult to admit your failures? If the answer is yes, think through your past trying to determine why this might be. _____

_____

_____

Question 8: Write a few sentences about this line from Step One in the *Twelve & Twelve*: "We perceive that only through utter defeat are we able to take our first steps toward liberation and strength."

_____

_____

_____

Reading Assignment 6, AA Big Book, Chapter 16

Question 9: Review this short paragraph from Part II, Chapter 16 below.

And acceptance is the answer to all my problems today. When I am disturbed, it is because I find some person, place, thing, or situation—some fact of my life—unacceptable to me, and I can find no serenity until I accept that person, place, thing, or situation as being exactly the way it is supposed to be at this moment. Nothing, absolutely nothing, happens in God's world by mistake. Until I could accept my alcoholism, I could not stay sober; unless I accept life completely on life's terms, I cannot be happy. I need to concentrate not so much on what needs to be changed in the world as on what needs to be changed in me and in my attitudes.

Think about how it applies to you and write at least three ways that you can use acceptance to improve your outlook on life.

1. _____

   _____

2. _____

   _____

3. _____

   _____

4. _____

   _____

5. _____

   _____

Worksheet B6: The What and When

Question 1: Use the list below; place a check in the box next to the different manifestations of addiction that appear in your life. If you are not sure if an item applies to you, ask for help from staff.

- ☐ Alcohol
- ☐ Benzodiazepines (Xanax, Valium, clonazepam, Ativan, etc.)
- ☐ Prescription opioids (oxycodone, hydrocodone, morphine, fentanyl, codeine, mitragynine (Kratom), oxymorphone, hydromorphone (Dilaudid), etc.)
- ☐ Illicit opioids (heroin, opium, and the like)
- ☐ Marijuana and marijuana products, including synthetic cannabinoids
- ☐ Cocaine
- ☐ Prescription stimulants (Adderall, Ritalin, and the like)
- ☐ Sleeping medications (zolpidem (Ambien), eszopiclone (Lunesta), zaleplon (Sonata))
- ☐ Methamphetamine
- ☐ "Bath Salts" (substituted cathinones)
- ☐ Hallucinogens (LSD, psilocybin, peyote, and the like)
- ☐ Ecstasy and related drugs (MDMA, MDA, and the like)
- ☐ Phencyclidine (PCP)
- ☐ Nicotine products (cigarettes, cigars, dip, and the like)
- ☐ Caffeine-containing products
- ☐ Other drugs (please describe) _____
- ☐ Compulsive sexual behavior
- ☐ Compulsive gambling
- ☐ Compulsive exercise
- ☐ Compulsive food bingeing or eating
- ☐ Compulsive food restriction (anorexia nervosa)
- ☐ Food bingeing, followed by purging via exercise, vomiting, laxatives, etc. (Bulimia Nervosa)
- ☐ Compulsive, non-job-related internet use
- ☐ Compulsive video game use
- ☐ Codependency—compulsive attention to or care taking of others that led to your own emotional or physical health problems
- ☐ A compulsive need to be in a romantic relationship
- ☐ Work addiction
- ☐ Compulsive shopping or spending
- ☐ Compulsive and destructive thrill seeking

☐ Hoarding or collecting seemingly useless items

☐ Other addiction behaviors, please describe _____

Question 2: Enter up to ten of the items you selected above in the first column below. Then, going from row to row, place a check mark in each box that defines the times in your life where your use occurred. Place a second check mark in the time period your use was the most intense or pervasive. When you have completed the time frame information, fill in the Rank column. Rank each of the addiction types from 1–5 (if you have five rows, 1–8 for eight rows, and so on). Your most prominent expression of your addiction should be a 1, your second most prominent a 2, and so on.

Addiction Manifestation	Rank	Age It Was Present in Your Life											
		<10	11–15	16–20	21–25	26–30	31–35	36–40	41–45	46–50	52–55	56–60	>60

Question 3: Looking at the above timeline, do you see any patterns where your addiction shifted from one manifestation to another? For example, you may have started smoking marijuana as a teenager, and then in your twenties you decreased your marijuana use dramatically, only to increase your alcohol use.

List how your addiction shifted from one manifestation to another in the table below.

At the approximate age of	My addiction shifted from	My addiction shifted more to

Question 4: Looking at the above timeline, do you see any patterns where two or more elements of your addiction seemed to coincide frequently? For example, "For a period of two years I used cocaine every time I drank alcohol." In the last column pick one or more reasons these elements of your addiction were combined. Use this list:

- To help with withdrawal
- To create a better high
- To cover up a more shameful addiction-related behavior
- To calm me down from another addiction-related behavior
- To disinhibit me so I could use another substance or engage in another behavior related to my addiction

At the approximate age of	I used . . .	I started using together or later switched to . . .	Describe one or more reasons why you think this occurred.

Question 5: Were there times in your life when it seemed that every aspect of your addiction stopped (whether you considered yourself in recovery or not)? List in the left column any times when this occurred. If you have ideas as to why you could stop, list these in the column to the right.

At the approximate age of	My addiction seemed to stop completely for		I think this happened because . . .
	Years	Months	

Addiction is a **progressive disease**. It progresses in several different manners. Think back on your struggle with addiction for a moment. Then answer the following questions.

Question 5a: Give three examples of how your use increased in amount over time. For alcohol and other drug use this is simply an increase in the amount used at a given sitting or the frequency with which you used. For a behavioral addiction, it is how much the behavior increased at a given time and how often you found yourself repeating this behavior.

1. _____

_____

2. _____

_____

3. _____

_____

Question 5b: Give three examples of how you lost the ability to control your use. Consider times when you tried to not use but used anyway or when you attempted to limit the time or extent of your use and could not. List them below.

1. _____

_____

2. _____

_____

3. _____

_____

Question 5c: Write down five examples of how your average using episode produced more extreme negative consequences to you. Consider your health, your self-esteem, your emotional stability, your financial stability, your ability to perform at your work or career, and difficulties with your family, friends, and loved ones.

1. _____

_____

_____

2. _____

_____

_____

3. _____

_____

_____

4. _____

_____

_____

5. _____

_____

_____

Worksheet B7: Your Addiction Life History

Welcome to your Addiction Life History. This is the most important assignment you will complete during your time in treatment. It is a large assignment with many pages. It is the only assignment in your workbook where you will use a separate pad of paper to record your thoughts. Your history will be a written narrative that lets other know who you are and more specifics about your disease history. Your Addiction Life History is completed in several steps. They are:

1. Your case manager will discuss with you when you should start your life history. Do not begin this task before you are ready.

2. Sit down and read this document in its entirety.

3. Complete the essay responses on a separate pad of paper. If you handwrite your answers, please make sure you or the staff can read your responses later.

4. When you have completed it, hand in your life history to your therapist or staff member. He or she will review your work. Your case manager may return your life history, asking for clarification in some areas. When it is complete, your case manager will allot time in Assignment Group.

5. Read your life history in Assignment Group. Your peers will provide support, ask questions, and relate their own similar experiences.

6. After you read and discuss your Addiction Life History, your case manager may ask you to revisit and revise certain sections and bring these changes back to Assignment Group.

Start working on this as soon as you receive this assignment from your case manager. This assignment will fill many pages. Do not expect to complete it in one evening or one day. Begin with the first section and quit if you feel overwhelmed, too upset, or very tired. These are all signs that your efforts on this assignment are paying off. We suggest you find a quiet spot where you can think, reflect, and maybe even talk to yourself.

In many ways, the Addiction Life History is the most important assignment you complete during your time in treatment. This assignment corrects the distortions AddictBrain manufactured inside your head. Some of these thoughts may be very real to you (e.g., "Alcohol helps me cope with stress."). You may be appalled by some of them (e.g., "Did I really drive my children around in the car when I was drunk?"). Nonetheless, you must correct, readjust, and realign your thoughts, responses, beliefs, and actions to build a solid recovery. This requires a thorough review of your life to date, focusing on how your addiction changed your core values and in doing so, changed who you were.

You may not want to face some events or emotions from your past. Push forward and write them down anyway. You may not want to disclose in group therapy everything you have written. Write it down now, you can make that decision later. Trust in this truth: "When your push the dark parts of your past out into a room with understanding peers, only then can you truly forgive yourself." The more thorough and fearless you are in completing your history, the better the outcome. When we ask for several examples, think through your potential responses until you find those that make you uneasy or upset. Write down these most difficult or painful responses in your life history.

When you relate events, spend some time painting the picture of what happened. Avoid answering questions with generalities (e.g., "I always went out drinking on Saturday night"). Instead, describe a specific incident that was scary, hurtful, or caused shame (e.g., "I remember one summer night five years ago when I . . . This night is hard to think about because I said the following cruel and uncalled-for things to . . ."). Be as exacting as you can be ("I used $300 of cocaine myself that evening." versus "We all bought cocaine and I used some."). Tie down the date of an event as best possible, even if you must go back and get it from an association ("It was the third year we lived in Cincinnati, we moved there in 1998, so it must have been around the spring of 2001"). You do not need to write down how you came up with the year and season in the example above but take the time to determine when important events occurred. If you are describing drug use be clear about what you took ("I took two 15 mg Xanax first then over the next four hours drank 6 to 8, 12 oz. beers," versus "I took some Xanax and got drunk.") Record your best recollection of what other people said; record their words if possible ("That was the night he told me, 'I wish I had never married you'"). Each of these techniques will help you remember events, as they truly happened, not how you wish you could remember them to avoid the pain. The basic principle is "AddictBrain loves vagueness, RecoveryMind demands clarity." The clearer you are about the difficult events of your past, the better equipped you will be to change the future.

Some of the questions ask you to describe important moments from your childhood, adolescent, young adult, and adult lives when you were criticized, belittled, led astray, abandoned, injured, or otherwise traumatized. We will make a special note of these sections. However, the bulk of this life and addiction history will examine how AddictBrain wreaked havoc, destroying your life and the lives of those around you. In instances where you were engaged in your addiction and were hurt, record how your illness damaged those around you rather than how others hurt you. Pay special attention in these areas not to blame ("I drank because my father left us when I was ten years old").

Traumatic events should be included in your life history. To help you remember such events later when you write out your addiction life history, write down five important life experiences that were especially traumatic for you below. After each one, fill out the details about each event. Write down why these events stand out and how you think they shaped your life.

1. _____

_____

_____

2. _____

_____

_____

3. _____

_____

_____

4. _____

_____

_____

5. _____

_____

_____

You may also want to write down the five most important events in your life that shaped it in a positive way.

1. _____

_____

_____

2. _____

_____

_____

3. _____

_____

_____

4. _____

_____

_____

5. _____

_____

_____

Your life history should be in an approximate chronological order. Put together important positive and negative events, including your addiction behaviors and its progression into this chronological story. Start with a bit of a backdrop if this is important, including family background, where you grew up, and where you lived. Describe fully the first time you drank or used substances or engaged in your behavioral addiction. Try to recall your age, the circumstances around the event, who you were with, and what you felt or experienced during this event. Move forward, weaving together your story. Remember to include how you felt about important events and how your actions affected those around you.

Please discuss important events in more detail. Do not just mention, "That was when my wife became really angry and moved out." Describe what was said, your feelings about the situation, how you coped, and the like. Describe your progression in your use with the most precise amounts and times as you can. Think about inflection points in your addiction, when and how did it accelerate or decelerate? The history should continue up until the present day.

Worksheet B8: Your First Step Summary

*Step One: We admitted we were powerless over our addiction—that our lives had
             become unmanageable.*

Bring this worksheet into Assignment Group on the day you are to present your Addiction Life History. After you present, the group will help you develop a synopsis, or abbreviated, first step. People who suffer from addiction disorders have difficulty seeing themselves. Members of your Assignment Group will help you list five ways in which you are powerless over your addiction and five ways your life has become unmanageable, based upon what they hear in your addiction life history. Write down the group responses below.

This brief, bulleted list of your own powerlessness and unmanageability will help you reinforce your commitment to the first step during the inevitable times in the future when recovery ambivalence reemerges. During those times, you might find it helpful to pull this form and read it to yourself. When you do so, the voices of your peers in the Assignment Group will come back to you, and you will find the peace that comes from accepting your addiction disorder.

I admit that I am powerless over my addiction. Five important and specific examples of my powerlessness that I acknowledge with the help of my peers are:

1. _____

   _____

   _____

2. _____

   _____

   _____

3. _____

   _____

   _____

4. _____
   _____
   _____

5. _____
   _____
   _____

I admit that my life has become unmanageable as a result of my addiction. Five important examples that help me know how my life is unmanageable are:

1. _____
   _____
   _____

2. _____
   _____
   _____

3. _____
   _____
   _____

4. _____
   _____
   _____

5. _____
   _____
   _____

Domain B: Progress Assessment Form

Basic Recovery: RecoveryMind Training

Domain B Recovery Skill	Date: Patient			Staff			Date: Patient			Staff			Date: Patient			Staff		
	B	I	C	B	I	C	B	I	C	B	I	C	B	I	C	B	I	C
Understands how to use Recovery Reflection as a self-monitoring and growth skill.																		
Is practicing Mindfulness Meditation or sound-based meditation two times daily.																		
Completed the Three by Five.																		
Understands and uses recovery literature and support group meetings.																		
Completed assigned readings in the Big Book (Chapters 1–4) and Step 1 in the 12 & 12.																		
Completed addiction history, presented in the Assignment Group and has responded with insight and subsequent personal growth.																		
Has "told on oneself" about current dishonesties and addictive thinking.																		
Has disclosed secrets about his or her past.																		
Has asked others for help addressing emotional unrest, denial, or other issues. Has asked others to hold him or her accountable in one or more recovery skills.																		
Is able to recognize and point out AddictBrain distortions of thought in **others**.																		
Is able to recognize and point out and correct AddictBrain distortions of thought in **self**.																		

This evaluation is completed by both the patient or client (self-assessment) and his or her therapist or staff members on this one form. After starting work on a skill, place the approximate start date in the in the provided column. The patient or client fills out the form first. A therapist or staff member performs the same evaluation, placing a check mark in each row that indicates progress in assigned Recovery Skills. This process may need to be repeated for a several times as work progresses in each domain.

A check mark in the **B** column signifies that work has begun. The **I** column should be checked if the patient is in an intermediate or midway through his or her work on this item, and the **C** column should be checked if the patient has made sufficient progress in the skill to move forward to his or her next task. Review and discussion of this form helps patients and therapists set clear treatment expectations and recovery goals.

Domain B: Recovery Basics Notes

1.   P. J. Carnes, R. E. Murray, and L. Charpentier. "Addiction Interaction Disorder." *Handbook of addictive disorders: A practical guide to diagnosis and treatment* (2004): 31–59.

2.   G. A. Marlatt, and N. Chawla. "Meditation and Alcohol Use." *South Med J* 100, no. 4 (2007): 451–53.

3.   B. E. Carlson, and H. Larkin. "Meditation as a Coping Intervention for Treatment of Addiction." *Journal of Religion & Spirituality in Social Work: Social Thought* 28, no. 4 (2009): 379–92.

4.   S. Bowen, N. Chawla, S. E. Collins, K. Witkiewitz, S. Hsu, J. Grow, S. Clifasefi, *et al.* "Mindfulness-Based Relapse Prevention for Substance Use Disorders: A Pilot Efficacy Trial." *Substance Abuse* 30, no. 4 (2009): 295-305.

5.   S. Bowen, N. Chawla, and G. Marlatt. *Mindfulness-Based Relapse Prevention for Addictive Behaviors: A Clinician's Guide.* Guilford Press, 2010.

6.   S. Bowen, K. Witkiewitz, S. L. Clifasefi, and et al. "Relative Efficacy of Mindfulness-Based Relapse Prevention, Standard Relapse Prevention, and Treatment as Usual for Substance Use Disorders: A Randomized Clinical Trial." *JAMA Psychiatry* 71, no. 5 (2014): 547-56.

7.   P. Chödrön. *How to Meditate : A Practical Guide to Making Friends with Your Mind.* Boulder, Colorado: Sounds True, 2013.

8.   Thich Nhat Hanh. *The Miracle of Mindfulness: An Introduction to the Practice of Meditation.* Boston: Beacon Press, 1976.

9.   J. Kornfield. *Meditation for Beginners.* New York: Bantam Books, 2005.

10.   T. Budzynski. "The Clinical Guide to Sound and Light." In *Stanford University*, edited by Stanford University. Palo Alto, CA, 2006.

11.   A. A. World Services. *Alcoholics Anonymous.* 4th ed. New York: A.A. World Services, 2013.

12.   Alcoholics Anonymous World Services. *Twelve Steps and Twelve Traditions.* New York: AA World Services, 2002.

Domain C: Emotional Awareness, and Resilience

Skills Groups, Assignments, Worksheets, and the Progress Assessment Form

Chapter Overview

Domain C is focused on our emotions and how they affect addiction diseases. Emotional experience is central to what it means to be a human being. Emotions color or flavor our daily experience, providing meaning and value to our existence. As much as they are a part of our joy, they are also at the core of our suffering. Most people spend considerable portion of their waking lives fighting battles with their internal emotional world. Some claim to be at peace with their interior emotional landscape. Others have learned, either consciously or unconsciously, to limit emotional responses in order to suppress painful feelings. Others displace or act out emotions to avoid having to sit uncomfortably in their presence. Indeed, it is the rare individual who can live his or her emotional life to the fullest, living in a world rich with emotion, complex and subtle, and at the same time remain centered and at peace.

Emotions are also closely related to an individual's character and temperament. In most cases, character and temperament is established prior to developing the addiction disorder. RecoveryMind Training asserts that AddictBrain subverts an individual's existing temperament and character to its own ends, exaggerating the maladaptive elements of personality to ensure its own survival.

AddictBrain also creates its own new emotions, alterations in character, and in behavioral responses. They become so ingrained that it is often difficult for people early in recovery to distinguish character traits or emotional responses that were present before the onset of an addiction disorder from those that develop as a result of the addiction itself. A client might express a desire to understand which attributes are acquired along the path into addiction from those that predate it—and are thus more at the core of his or her being. This is at best a fool's errand.

Instead, in Domain C I focus on realigning the client's personality to make healthy responses. When the client is happy and healthy, the quest to differentiate emotional origins seems less important. Building a new personality is one of the most important outcomes of consistent attendance at AA meetings. For example, after consistent attendance at AA (or its sister organizations) you might hear a client say, "I've adopted an 'attitude of gratitude." Alternatively, you may hear a person in recovery say things like "That was my alcoholic side (addict side) acting out again. Pay it no mind."

Emotions were first postulated as being basic biological events by Charles Darwin.[1] It also appears that emotions are hard-wired and universal; Ekman reported that the facial expression of emotions is universal across cultures.[2,3] More recent research suggest we recognize the emotions of others and our own emotions by processing subtle facial movements.[4,5] Psychologists have developed several systems for categorizing emotions. One such categorization suggests we have seven fundamental emotions, expressed in the same manner by all human beings and may even be universal to higher animals. This system may not jibe with current brain studies, but it is helpful to simplify our understanding of our emotions. This system postulates that certain basic emotions exist and that they are:

1. **Happiness/Joy**: A natural smile produces wrinkles around the eyes whereas the social smile only engages the mouth. In a genuine smile, the area between the eyebrow and the eye decreases, and the cheeks raise, producing crow's feet.

2. **Surprise**: Involves the raising of the eyebrows and eyelids, and sometimes a dropping of the jaw.

3. **Contempt**: This is identified by a half smile, a half dimple, and/or a one-sided lip raise.

4. **Sadness**: The most reliable indicator of sadness is the raising of the inner corners of the eyebrows.

5. **Fear**: Fear is like surprise; however, the brow lowers in fear.

6. **Disgust**: Recognized most by the wrinkling of the nose or the raising of the upper lip.

7. **Anger**: The main ingredients of anger include the lowering of the eyebrows, raising and tightening of the eyelids. This can also include any number of other factors such as clenching the jaw, gritting teeth, or tightening the lips.

Beyond these basic emotions, there are many schemes for outlining emotional states. It may be helpful to organize and interconnect feelings using a system[6] developed by Robert Plutchik, shown diagrammatically below.

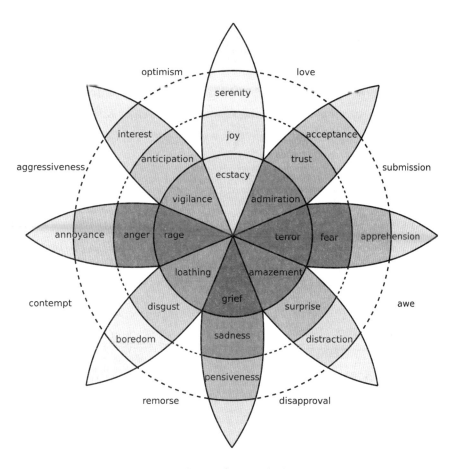

Figure C1 – Plutchik's Wheel of Emotions

Emotions, by their very nature, feel as if they are the core of the thing we call "me." Unlike thoughts or ideas, emotions cannot be experienced as originating outside of oneself. Even when we feel someone else's emotions through empathy, we recognize the feelings of others as they resonate similar feelings in our own mind. AddictBrain uses this "me-ness," when it hijacks the limbic area (the brain's emotional center) causing confusion between the individual and his or her disease. During addiction or in the first several years of recovery, individuals commonly experience emotional states either caused or manipulated by AddictBrain. The hold AddictBrain has on our limbic area is intricate and tenacious. When an AddictBrain-generated emotion occurs, it feels as if it comes from the center of personal experience, the core of our being, the thing we call "me." As you can well imagine, this wreaks havoc on the addicted individual as he or she battles his or her disease. Displacing this hold demands a consistent and determined effort. Empirical research shows that some techniques help emotional resilience more than others.[7] RecoveryMind teaches patients to be wary of their "emotional truth. We ask them to wonder if a particular feeling or belief (held in place by its emotional veracity) " . . . could it not be your own, but rather a foreign AddictBrain, pushing you toward its agenda of keeping you sick?"

In Domain C, the exercises focus on three areas: helping patients experience their emotional world; preventing that emotional experience from being destructive to self or others; and differentiating one's true emotions from those of AddictBrain. To do this well, all patients begin with a solid foundation in preliminary skills, including:

- Recognizing and accurately naming emotional states in self
- Recognizing and accurately naming emotional states in others
- Experiencing and "leaning into" difficult emotions—to experience emotions to their fullest
- Tolerating the distress produced by all emotions—both pleasant and unpleasant—with minimal projection, acting out, denial, or intellectualization

Some clients will not require work on these skills; others may need extensive work in this area. Only make assignments in these areas when a given individual needs work in that area. Once these skills are validated as present or improved through exercises in Domain C, a client can move on to practice:

- Experiencing emotional states without digressing into addictive chemicals and behaviors
- Questioning whether a given emotional state acts in the service of AddictBrain or RecoveryMind
- Recognizing common emotional ploys that AddictBrain uses to drive relapse

We all know individuals who are not addicted nor in recovery who are completely lacking in such emotional skills. According to RecoveryMind Training, "Individuals with addiction do not have the luxury of going through life without knowing and at least making an unsteady peace with their feelings." A rich recovery occurs when one fully embraces his or her emotional life. Relapse can and will occur if those in recovery do not develop a deeper understanding of their feelings.

Domain C has four Skills Groups:
- C1) Emotional Recognition: Identifying emotions in self and others
- C2) Learning to "surf" uncomfortable emotions
- C3) Default emotions role-play
- C4) Role-play feeling states driven by AddictBrain

There are three Assignment Group tasks in Domain C:

C1) Read conclusions from the Emotional Acceptance Worksheet aloud and receive feedback

C2) Read the Default Emotions Worksheet aloud and consider group feedback.

C3) Read aloud the Emotional Games of AddictBrain Worksheet and receive feedback.

Remember that mental exploration of feelings and writing that exploration down on paper are components of a cognitive exercise; at its core, this is thinking about emotions, not experiencing them. The bulk of work in this domain must occur in a therapeutic setting where participants express emotions, have them recognized and validated by others, and are encouraged to express them to their fullest while simultaneously preventing a self-destructive reaction (e.g., acting out through using). Completing Domain C worksheets must be paired with expression of feeling states in Skills Groups and exploring issues that arise from this work in a Process Group.

There are four Worksheets in Domain C:

C1) The **Emotion Acceptance Worksheet**. This worksheet helps patients differentiate emotions that they are comfortable with from those that are uncomfortable. This worksheet then explores maladaptive patterns with these uncomfortable emotions.

C2) The **My Default Emotion Worksheet**. Patients review the Emotion Acceptance Worksheet looking for feelings they unconsciously mutate from difficult emotional states into emotions they are more comfortable experiencing. An example might be shifting anger into guilt. These are called *default emotions*. Then the patient looks to see if any of his or her default emotions drive his or her addiction illness.

C3) The **Emotional Games of AddictBrain Worksheet**. This worksheet uses the knowledge gained in previous worksheets, Assignment Groups and related discussions to increase awareness of the way AddictBrain hijacks his or her own emotional states to further entrench the addicted state. This concept may be difficult for some patients. If so, it should be approached with an attitude of exploration rather than certitude.

C4) The **Stories from My Life Worksheet**. Each patient records three especially poignant stories from his or her life. Then writes down his or her age, the setting, who was involved and what happened. With this worksheet, the author is not searching for specific emotions but rather recording significant events so these events can be explored later in Process Group; the group helps him or her using the skills he or she has learned previously in this domain.

Domain C: Skills Groups

Skills Group C1: Emotional Recognition

To those of us who attend or conduct psychotherapy, it may be surprising to learn that many people walk our planet unaware or confused about what they feel. Some may bottle up emotions until they become jumbled up inside, their feelings eventually tangling into a Gordian knot. Some may have learned as children to suppress or "bottle up" feelings. Such individuals describe "stress or pressure," rather than specific feeling states. Some may swap an "unacceptable" emotion for an "acceptable" one. The classic example from many cultures is "boys don't cry" (they get angry) and "anger is unladylike" (they develop depression and guilt). Some may vent all emotional states through a default emotion, such as anger. Some may not recognize their emotional state and act out their feelings instead. Some may constantly project feelings onto others seeing the world as hostile when they are angry, threatening when they themselves want to attack. Others view those around them as fragile when they themselves are in a vulnerable state. A few may be apparently barren of emotions, a state known as *alexithymia*, the inability to name or know feelings.[8] When we bypass, convert, suppress, or repress our emotions, we lose contact with self and become more vulnerable to addiction and addiction relapse. When we accept and sit with our emotions for a time, we develop a deeper understanding and patience. AddictBrain cannot use our emotional awkwardness to trigger relapse or promote continued use. This defines the work at hand in Domain C.

Skills Group C1 has two parts. The group begins with a brief relaxation exercise (leader's choice). The leader may connect physical experience with feeling states using the following exercise.

> The leader asks patients to scan their bodies, noticing any physical discomfort or ill ease. Is there tension in the legs? What does this feel like? Is there pain in the lower back? What does it want to do? Does the head feel full? The leader asks a participant to volunteer the physical feeling. The leader asks him, "If this part of the body could speak what feelings would it express? The leader gently discourages digressions about physical pain ("I know that is an issue for you, but we need to focus on our emotions in this session"). The leader deepens the feeling by asking more about the feeling: why are you here now, "Are there more words to describe the feeling? Is it connected with any past event?" Members of the group also participate by asking questions, "Does this hurt ever make you angry?" They also observe, ask questions, and provide feedback, "You use the word irritated, but your face looks sad. Is there sadness to this feeling?" The leader changes protagonist by asking, "Who else can share a feeling trapped in their body?"

Another way of exploring feelings is to ask about small acting-out behaviors.

The leader asks group members to think of a surprising behavior from the past several days. For this group, it is best to stay away from heavy events. A participant may volunteer with "I had decided to cut out all desserts this week, and I was doing well with this until yesterday when at lunch I grabbed a large piece of pie in the cafeteria." The group asks the protagonist what she was feeling at that moment or in the period leading up to lunch. Group members help the protagonist with the incident by asking questions, such as "You were talking about your husband in group therapy just before lunch, could that be related?" The group explores multiple possibilities, assiduously avoiding pat answers that led to such events.

In the second part of this group, a protagonist is identified who has completed Worksheet C3. The protagonist reads from the *Stories from My Life* worksheet. Other members listen to the story and describe what past emotions the protagonist is expressing in his or her story. This leads to a stop and start reading of the story that the leader modulates appropriately, balancing increased understanding with repeated interruption of the story content. When the assignment reading is complete, members attempt to identify feelings the protagonist experienced while *telling* the story. The emotions may be the same or may wind up being different. When a group member describes a feeling in the story and this matches the patient's emotional state, group members validate the identifier (use "yes" or "that's it"). When the protagonist states the feedback is incorrect, discussion ensues. Did the feedback misjudge what the protagonist was feeling? Or, did the protagonist misinterpret his or her own feelings, i.e., the read by another was accurate and the protagonist has unrecognized emotions that the other members are sensing.

If time permits, the leader picks one of the stories and acts it out in psychodrama. The protagonist is encouraged to express emotions that were withheld in the past. If trained in more advanced experiential techniques, the leader can use doubling, role reversal, or protagonist mirroring to explore past emotions. The leader cautiously connects past hurt with present vulnerability to relapse when appropriate.

This Skills Group builds emotional awareness for all its members. Skills developed here decrease the vulnerability to relapse and prepare the patient for additional work in Domains E and F.

Skills Group C2: Surfing Uncomfortable Emotions

The concept of "surfing" uncomfortable emotions, urges, or cravings was first described by G. Alan Marlatt, PhD. In fact, most elements of relapse prevention training are based upon his work and of his mentees.[9] Apparently, Dr. Marlatt was working with an individual in early recovery whose first love was the sport of surfing. He developed the concept of surfing the cravings of addiction with this patient.[10] Dialectical Behavioral Therapy (DBT) adapted this skill to help patients manage the uncomfortable aspects of strong emotions. RecoveryMind training uses the skill of "surfing urges" twice—once in Group C2 in dealing, sitting with, and managing emotional states and later on in Domain F when building relapse prevention skills. This Skills Group is based upon the work of Bowen, et al.[11] and Larimer, et al.[12] It starts with a ten-minute introduction, during which time the leader describes the techniques and the desired outcome.

Start the group with a brief introductory lecture delineating the following material.

> Everyone has discomforting emotions. Most of us try to manage feelings by avoiding them or fighting back. Paradoxically, such mental efforts only reinforce the strength of urges and painful emotions. This is like feeding a stray cat. Once you start feeding the animal (by not properly owning the feeling state), you can count on it to return again and again. It is difficult to sit with certain emotions; we use an unconsciously acquired automatic response, such as acting out, using denial, repression, or suppression. Later the urge or emotion sneaks up, and, before we know it, we are acting on it—long before we realize the danger. As we learn how to be comfortable with difficult emotional states, they are more likely to surface, be given their due, worked through, and let be. We recognize such a difficult emotion, allow it to sit within us, and then watch it disappear. Being mindful and noticing emotional states and urges to act on them provides us with the time and space to prevent knee-jerk actions, which are almost always the wrong course to take.

> In addition, feelings have a sense of urgency attached to them. They command our attention. However, the worst thing powerful and uncomfortable feelings can do is make us feel them. They are not threatening to us in any other way. Our reactions to feelings produce the most harm. Urges by nature have an inevitable quality as well. "If I don't scratch that itch, it will keep on building until I have to scratch!" Despite the quality of inevitability, urges do come and go. It is best to think of this feature as a trick or a fraud. We will learn how to watch an urge wax and wane. This is the most important talent to learn in this Skills Group.

The Practice of Feeling or "Urge Surfing"

Start by telling patients that this is skills practice. There is no grade, no pressure to perform. Explain that some people will take to this skill easily; others may have problems with it.

After this introduction, you begin the practice. The instructions are as follows:

> If you have judgmental thoughts during this exercise, let them go. Take a deep breath in and out. In doing so, come into the here and now. Find a comfortable, but quietly alert, posture. Let your eyes close slowly and gently. Notice the room around you. If you are not experiencing any uncomfortable feelings or urges, scan through your recent past to pull up such an emotion. Or, refocus on a current urge or feeling that troubles you. Commit yourself to stay with this feeling without reacting, suppressing, or thinking it away. See what it is like. Watch as the feeling or urge increases or decreases in intensity over time. Do not try to change it or manipulate it in any fashion; simply watch it. Breathe into the feeling. Inhale it with your breath. Recall the thoughts that come with this emotion. Acknowledge your reactions to this emotion (*It scares me, I feel a need to move, I want to cry, and the like.*) Stay with the feeling without trying to control it, push it away, or take any action at all. Again watch it increase or decrease in intensity. Imagine the feeling like a wave that rises. During the rising, notice how it seems as if it will go on forever. Stay with the feeling, noticing it without reacting. Stay calm and breathe the emotion in slowly. After a time, watch the wave crest and fall. Stay present and surf, riding the wave of emotion.

Remember to talk patients through this process with a calm, slow voice. When a sufficient time has elapsed for each member to practice this skill, instruct the participants to return to the room. Then ask group members to return to the room and open their eyes slowly.

The leader asks one or more of the following questions to encourage discussion.

- Were you able to pull up a strong urge or emotion?
- Could you sit with the emotion without trying to suppress or push it away?
- Could you surf the urge?
- Did it crest or just build?
- What else did you notice?
- Did anyone want to get up and bolt out of the room?

After a period of discussion, make sure to instruct participants to practice urge surfing. When they do, they should be in a safe environment where they cannot act out the feeling or urge. Patients should be told that they should not act on any urge or feeling for at least twenty-four hours after practicing urge surfing; they should do so only after discussing their proposed action with a staff member or in group therapy.

Skills Group C3: Default Emotions Role Play

The leader begins this group with a brief description of how each of us learned in our childhood which emotions we could and could not express. When we were younger, there are often messages from parental figures that certain emotions were taboo and should not be felt. Later in life, as these feelings arise, we have little practice in sitting with them, naturally expressing them and working them through. Such feelings are suppressed, repressed, or acted out in self-destructive behaviors.

In this Skills Group, patients who have completed Worksheets C1 and C2 act as the protagonist in a skill-building exercise. This role-play uses a technique from psychodrama called *mirroring* or *doubling* to help each patient understand his or her relationship with feelings. The group leader should be trained in this technique before attempting it with patients. A protagonist is selected; she sits at the front of the audience and picks an individual to be her double. Several other family members from the childhood or current nuclear family (or close friends) are enrolled. Reading off their C1 Worksheet, the protagonist directs her double to act out feelings noted from the first column (the emotions that "are expressed easily or often") to an appropriate auxiliary. The protagonist gently corrects the expression of these feelings until they feel accurate. Next, the protagonist does this same process for feelings in the second column (Difficulty Expressing) paying special attention to directing such emotions to the correct enrolled auxiliary.

The last and more important part of this group comes from Worksheet C2. The protagonist directs her double to express a default emotion from Worksheet C2. Standing behind her double, she watches this feeling being expressed. She then whispers the true hidden or repressed emotions (the ones that were defaulted), instructing the double to express them one at a time. The protagonist views the scene from multiple vantage points, standing behind her double, beside the scene and behind the auxiliary who acts as the feeling recipient, the protagonist integrates every aspect of the emotional experience. They recognize what it is like to express or receive the target emotion. Time permitting, the protagonist has the auxiliaries to role-play past events, noticing that difficult emotions have no inherent good or bad qualities. They are as important and valid as "acceptable" emotions.

At the conclusion of the scene, participants disenroll one by one. Everyone in the room participates in an open discussion of the experience. Non-active group members are encouraged to relate the scene to their own life. If time permits, another participant comes forward and a new scene with a different protagonist unfolds.

Skills Group C4: Role-Play AddictBrain Feeling States

This Skills Group repeats the structure of Skills Group C3 but focuses on feelings that are related to addiction. A protagonist who has already completed Worksheet C2 is selected. He or she asks a group member to be his or her double.[13] He or she then asks other group members to enroll as important figures from his or her past or current life (family, friends, and coworkers). The double acts out emotions from Column 4 (Would Use to Feel). The protagonist watches the expression of these emotions, gently correcting his or her double with the help of the group leader. The protagonist also instructs other enrolled members of the scene to respond accurately based upon his or her history. Through the course of the scene, the protagonist learns how such feelings were related to past events. The protagonist develops a broader experience with trigger feeling states.

When these feeling are well explored, the scene moves on to act out emotions from Column 5 of Worksheet C1. When expressed, the protagonist learns to accept and normalize the difficult parts of these feeling states. As in Skills Group C3, once complete, the entire group discusses their emotional experiences. Sharing is encouraged; advice giving is discouraged. At the end of each discussion segment, the group leader may provide a brief summary and analysis of the scene.

If the protagonist has completed Worksheet C3 (The Emotional Games of AddictBrain), the scene can be very clearly mapped onto the psychodrama stage. The protagonist enrolls an auxiliary to amplify the uncomfortable emotion. Additional auxiliaries might play the qualities of the target emotion. When the protagonist has a true scene, the leader has them enroll AddictBrain, who strolls in casually, but in control, telling the protagonist that they "have a right to all this grief, after all look what you have been through!" The feeling auxiliaries reiterate the feeling "You are **so** sad." The AddictBrain auxiliary agrees, adding, "You deserve to use a little cocaine to feel better." If the loss is enrolled, it provides a different vantage point: "I know you miss me, but I want you to be happy and in recovery. You can honor my memory best by being healthy and in recovery!"

Domain C: Assignment Group Tasks

Assignment Group Task C1

In this Assignment Group task, one or more patients bring their Emotion Acceptance (Worksheet C1) to the group for discussion. Rather than read the entire list of feelings, the protagonist goes through his or her list one column at a time (i.e., start with describing emotions that are expressed easily or often), reading and commenting briefly on the emotions in this list pausing for feedback at the end of the column. The leader may ask the reader to note important emotions if the list is overly inclusive. Group participants are encouraged to suggest other emotions based upon their understanding of the individual, ask for examples, and ask about specific incidents from the protagonist's past. Once the first column has been completed, the exercise proceeds through each of the five columns of the worksheet. The group can often provide the most help with the third column—emotions that are difficult to experience in others. The protagonist may need to revise his or her worksheet, using feedback provided during this assignment. When appropriate, the leader guides additional discussion. Others in the group are encouraged to rethink their relationship with emotions based upon the ensuing discussion.

Assignment Group Task C2

In this Assignment Group task, the protagonist reads his or her completed answers to the Default Emotions Worksheet. This is a brief exercise with group feedback that varies, depending upon the protagonist's insight. Feedback from others in the group often provides additional insight ("It seems that no matter what happens when you talk with your spouse, you wind up angry.") This assignment and the C1 Assignment should be completed prior to the protagonist taking these worksheets to Skills Group C3.

Assignment Group Task C3

In this group the assigned protagonist reads the Emotional Games of AddictBrain (Worksheet C3) to the group. The protagonist reads each important emotion and the qualities that are the most difficult about that feeling and begins exploring how AddictBrain uses strong emotions (both positive and negative) to keep him or her sick. Often the patient may not be able to see this third part, but his or her peers will often see it clearly. Most clients are resistant to acknowledging that AddictBrain hijacks their feelings. This is especially true for feeling states that seem "justified"—such as the hostility directed at a soon-to-be recently divorced husband or wife or the grief of a parent who has lost a child in the past. They deserve validation about such emotions. The leader follows group validation with "How could AddictBrain use this against you?" For those who are highly reactive, it is best to frame this assignment as an "exploration of possibilities" rather than established fact.

Clients who observe this assignment may get more out of it than the protagonist. They will see the protagonist's blindness and resistance clearly. The leader should encourage such individuals to express their opinion, shifting focus briefly to increase the opinion-giver's insight into his or her own hijacked emotions.

Assignment Group Task C4

Assignment Group Task C4 involves reading the contents of Worksheet C4. This group assignment may not always be completed. It is often set aside for later psychotherapy work in emotionally fragile patients. The therapist reviews the completion, scanning for issues that could "flip the switch" of emotional insight (a client who was traumatized by controlling and intrusive parents and who subverts a center's schedule or simple recovery rules in a misdirected, unconscious need to overthrow past parental control). In such a case, reviewing the past event with group validation and empathy is meaningful, especially if such a patient is able to connect it with difficulties in accepting necessary tasks in recovery.

Domain C: Emotional Resilience Worksheets

Overview of Worksheets

The worksheets in this domain teach basic emotional skills for a solid recovery. Worksheets in this domain help patients recognize their feeling states and teach basic skills in managing emotions. Some patients may need additional skills in emotions management. For those individuals, I recommend more rigorous work in Dialectical Behavior Therapy.

There are four worksheets in Domain C. The therapist assigns one or more worksheets based upon patient needs in the area covered by the worksheet. A patient with limited connection with his or her emotions would be assigned Worksheet C1. A patient who seems to ride one emotion over and over, regardless of situation, may need to focus on Worksheet C2. Most individuals who have been struggling with addiction for some time have been victimized by AddictBrain's subversive control of their emotions. In these cases, completing either or both Worksheets C1 and C2 should come first, then work should commence on Worksheet C3. Finally, many clients or patients who have had painful or traumatic events in their past should be considered for Worksheet C4. Remember, RecoveryMind Training provides multiple therapeutic opportunities through the Skills Groups, assignments, and Worksheets. A skilled therapist or treatment team selects a subset of these exercises for a given client or patient, matching his or her needs with the tools provided here. The worksheet tools in Domain C are:

C1) The **Acceptance of Emotions** Worksheet. This worksheet helps patients differentiate the emotions that they are comfortable and uncomfortable experiencing. For the uncomfortable emotions, it goes on to explore maladaptive patterns with these emotions.

C2) The **Default Emotions** Worksheet. Patients review the Acceptance of Emotion Worksheet looking for feelings they unconsciously mutate from difficult emotional states into emotions they are more comfortable experiencing. An example might be shifting anger into guilt. These are called *default emotions*. Then, the patient looks to see if any of his or her default emotions promote addiction or sabotage recovery.

C3) The **Emotional Games of AddictBrain** Worksheet. Building on the exploration of the first two worksheets, Worksheet C3 explores how AddictBrain uses emotions for its own agenda. Here, patients will discover how their addiction wants to keep them depressed or angry or how AddictBrain thrives on repressed anger or unmet longing.

C4) The **Stories from My Life** Worksheet. Each patient records three stories from his or her life that were especially poignant. He or she writes down the age, setting, who was involved, and what happened. The client should not specifically state emotions that occurred during these incidents although they are implied in the stories. The emotions will be explored when the stories are read in Assignment Group and may be used in Skills Group C4.

Worksheet C1: Acceptance of Emotions

There are many ways of categorizing our emotions. Many anthropologists and neuroscientists agree that there are seven primary emotions, **Happiness / Joy**, **Surprise**, **Contempt**, **Sadness**, **Fear**, **Disgust**, and **Anger**. This short list does not come close to the varied experiences and sensations we feel from our emotions. Each of us recognizes and experiences the myriad emotions in different degrees and manners. However, once expressed, they are usually recognizable by others. In recovery we need to learn how to know and express our emotions to their fullest extent without jeopardizing others. When we suppress, act out, or subvert one feeling for another, we become ill. Our loved ones, friends, and coworkers are also affected. AddictBrain loves it when we circumvent our hurt and loss, suppress our anger, or repress our joy. Each of these actions fuels the fire of addiction and makes it harder to gain and retain recovery.

The exercises in Domain C are important to start you on your recovery journey. If you have depression, anxiety, or other psychological or psychiatric disease, work in Domain C is especially important for you.

Question 1: To complete question 1, work through the entire list five separate times. This exercise may take some time. Pace yourself, complete twenty to thirty emotions at a sitting, take a break, and return to it when you can. Do not rush through this exercise; be thoughtful about your answers. Complete this worksheet in the following order:

1. To begin this worksheet, go down the list of feelings and place one check mark in the column ① next to any feeling you can easily express or find yourself feeling or expressing often. Place two check marks in column ① if that feeling occurs very often. You should not place check marks next to every feeling you experience. Be selective and think about this item as you complete it. Concentrate on the emotions that seem to be more frequent or stronger for you and mark them in this part of the exercise.

2. Next, return to the top of the list and go down it again, placing one check mark in the column ② next to any emotion you have difficulty feeling or expressing. Place two check marks in column ② if you have extreme difficulty expressing the corresponding emotion. There may be any number of emotions you mark or do not mark here as well. Mark only those emotions that apply to you in this manner.

3. Return to the top and go down the list a third time, placing one check mark in the column ③ if you have difficulty being around someone else when he or she is having or expressing the given emotion. Place two check marks in column ③ if you will do anything to get away from someone who is expressing this emotion.

4. Return to the top of the list to relate feeling states to your addiction. Go through the list a fourth time, entering one check mark in column ④ next to a feeling you would use to

stimulate that emotion. Place two check marks in column ④ if this was an important feeling you used to stimulate.

5. Finally, return to the top of the list to consider feeling states you would try to escape or suppress by using (engaging in your addiction). Place one check mark in the column ⑤ next to an emotion you would use alcohol or other drugs or engage in a behavioral or food addiction to try to escape from or suppress. Place two check marks in column ⑤ if this was a very important feeling (one that would produce an extremely strong need to push away by using substances).

Feeling or Emotion	① I express this feeling easily or often	② I have difficulty feeling or expressing . . .	③ It is difficult being around others when they are feeling . . .	④ I would "use" to feel this emotion . . .	⑤ I would "use" to avoid this feeling . . .
Fear					
apprehension					
dread					
foreboding					
frightened					
mistrust					
panic					
petrified					
scared					
suspicious					
terror					
wary					
worried					
Annoyance					
aggravated					
dismayed					
disgruntled					
displeased					
exasperated					
frustrated					
impatient					
irritated					
critical					
irked					

Feeling or Emotion	① I express this feeling easily or often	② I have difficulty feeling or expressing . . .	③ It is difficult being around others when they are feeling . . .	④ I would "use" to feel this emotion . . .	⑤ I would "use" to avoid this feeling . . .
Anger					
enraged					
furious					
incensed					
indignant					
irate					
livid					
outraged					
resentful					
animosity					
Aversion					
appalled					
contempt					
disgust					
dislike					
hate					
horrified					
hostile					
repulsed					
ambivalent					
Confused					
baffled					
bewildered					
dazed					

Feeling or Emotion	① I express this feeling easily or often	② I have difficulty feeling or expressing . . .	③ It is difficult being around others when they are feeling . . .	④ I would "use" to feel this emotion . . .	⑤ I would "use" to avoid this feeling . . .
hesitant					
lost					
mystified					
perplexed					
puzzled					
torn					
Emotions of Disconnection					
alienated					
aloof					
apathetic					
bored					
cold					
detached					
distant					
distracted					
indifferent					
numb					
removed					
uninterested					
skeptical					
selfish					
withdrawn					
ashamed					

Feeling or Emotion	① I express this feeling easily or often	② I have difficulty feeling or expressing . . .	③ It is difficult being around others when they are feeling . . .	④ I would "use" to feel this emotion . . .	⑤ I would "use" to avoid this feeling . . .
Embarrassed					
chagrin					
flustered					
guilt					
mortified					
self-conscious					
embarrassed					
stupid					
beat					
Fatigue					
burnt out					
depleted					
exhausted					
lethargic					
listless					
sleepy					
tired					
weary					
worn out					
agony					
Pain and Loss					
anguish					
bereaved					
devastated					

Feeling or Emotion	① I express this feeling easily or often	② I have difficulty feeling or expressing . . .	③ It is difficult being around others when they are feeling . . .	④ I would "use" to feel this emotion . . .	⑤ I would "use" to avoid this feeling . . .
grief					
heartbroken					
hurt					
lonely					
miserable					
regretful					
rejected					
remorseful					
depressed					
Sadness and Sorrow					
dejected					
despair					
despondent					
disappointed					
discouraged					
disheartened					
forlorn					
gloomy					
heavyhearted					
hopeless					
melancholy					
unhappy					
wretched					
anxious					

Feeling or Emotion	① I express this feeling easily or often	② I have difficulty feeling or expressing . . .	③ It is difficult being around others when they are feeling . . .	④ I would "use" to feel this emotion . . .	⑤ I would "use" to avoid this feeling . . .
Tension and Anxiety					
cranky					
distressed					
distraught					
edgy					
fidgety					
frazzled					
irritable					
jittery					
nervous					
overwhelmed					
restless					
stressed out					
fragile					
Vulnerable					
guarded					
helpless					
bashful					
insecure					
leery					
reserved					
sensitive					
submissive					
insignificant					

Feeling or Emotion	① I express this feeling easily or often	② I have difficulty feeling or expressing . . .	③ It is difficult being around others when they are feeling . . .	④ I would "use" to feel this emotion . . .	⑤ I would "use" to avoid this feeling . . .
shaky					
inadequate					
inferior					
weak					
foolish					
envious					
Yearning					
jealous					
longing					
nostalgic					
pining					
wistful					
Joyful					
excited					
energetic					
playful					
creative					
aware					
sexy					
daring					
fascinated					
stimulated					
amused					
extravagant					

Feeling or Emotion	① I express this feeling easily or often	② I have difficulty feeling or expressing . . .	③ It is difficult being around others when they are feeling . . .	④ I would "use" to feel this emotion . . .	⑤ I would "use" to avoid this feeling . . .
delighted					
Self-confident					
powerful					
respected					
proud					
appreciated					
hopeful					
important					
faithful					
cheerful					
satisfied					
valuable					
worthwhile					
intelligent					
confident					
Peaceful					
peaceful					
content					
thoughtful					
loving					
trusting					
nurturing					
relaxed					
responsive					

Feeling or Emotion	① I express this feeling easily or often	② I have difficulty feeling or expressing . . .	③ It is difficult being around others when they are feeling . . .	④ I would "use" to feel this emotion . . .	⑤ I would "use" to avoid this feeling . .
serene					
sentimental					
thankful					

This feeling list was adapted and expanded from original work by the Center for Nonviolent Communication.

The original list: Copyright © 2005 by the Center for Nonviolent Communication.

Question 2: Return to the list above reviewing columns ② and ③ for emotions that you find especially difficult. Try to connect this difficulty to past events or childhood experiences. If you can relate one or more feelings to the past, place them in the list below.

Difficult emotion above	Past event or childhood experience to which this might be related

Worksheet C2: Default Emotions

Most of us work to control our feelings, allowing access to some emotions over others. In Worksheet C1, you built a list of emotions that you were less comfortable experiencing or expressing when alone or in the company of others. In this worksheet, you will consider emotions you express more often. On face value, you may think you express these emotions more often simply because that is the way you feel. This could be partly true. However, many people also unconsciously (or even consciously) divert the energy from one feeling (that is less acceptable or tolerable) to a more comfortable feeling state. I call this a "Default Emotion." A *default emotion* is a "cover" for less comfortable feelings.

Everyone has one or more default emotion(s) that they express more often and with more ease. Your friends and family may notice them saying, "That Jerry, he is always so sarcastic." This creates problems if the energy of uncomfortable emotional states is repeatedly expressed through alternates. First your friends and family will always be responding in an unsatisfactory manner; you wind up feeling chronically misunderstood (often without knowing why). Second you become confused about what you truly experience and feel. Thirdly, and most critical, the "disconnect" between your deeper feelings and the expression of those feelings create an emotional rift. AddictBrain exploits and resides in this rift. It widens and deepens it. The resulting emotional discord fuels addiction. Therefore, it is critical to interrupt default emotions whenever possible for a more meaningful recovery.

Question 1: Review the feeling list in Worksheet C2, looking for one or more feelings you seem to feel and express often. Then ask you family and friends for emotions or emotional attitudes you seem most often to carry about you or express. Weed through the possibilities to create a short list of one to three default emotions. Record them below.

Feelings or emotional states that I seem to express the most often are _____

_____

_____

_____

Question 2: Go through the list again looking for emotions you rarely display. Recall and pay special attention to any emotions that you were discouraged or prohibited from expressing in your childhood. Consider whether any of these difficult or forbidden emotions may be converted to the default emotion(s) listed above. You may feel like you are guessing when you fill out this section, and that's okay. This exercise is an exploration. If you think it is possible, record it below.

Sometimes when I show this emotion	I might be expressing the emotional energy of this (or these) emotions

Question 3: If there is one emotion I seem to express more than any other, it is _____

And the emotions I rarely if ever express are _____

_____

_____

Worksheet C3: The Emotional Games of AddictBrain

AddictBrain is constantly plotting inside your head, hoping to sustain your addiction or to goad you into relapse. It does this by changing your perspective, rearranging priorities, creating cravings, and modifying your emotions. This worksheet helps you look at how your feelings and emotional state place you at risk for relapse.

Question 1: Retrieve Worksheet C1 and review the feelings and emotions there, paying special attention to any correlation between feeling states that you marked in columns ② or ③ that also show up in columns ④ or ⑤. Use the example in the first row below to help guide how you complete this question.

Make a note of the most important of these emotions in the column ① below. Next, make a note of the qualities of these emotions in column ②. Spend some time thinking about the emotions you record in this list and describe what it feels like to have them occur. You can start with the qualities from the emotions list column headings in Worksheet C1 (i.e., ① Expressed easily, ② Difficulty feeling, ③ Difficulty being around others who are expressing these emotions, ④ Would use to feel, and ⑤ Would use to avoid feeling) and add other qualities to these emotions to better qualify them (e.g., seems like it is always there, sneaks up and surprises me, I wake up at night with this feeling, it feels heavy in my chest, feeling good makes me anxious, and such). Lastly, fill out column ③ below, looking for how AddictBrain could use this emotion against you. Repeat this for each of the important emotions you list from Worksheet C1.

① An important emotion from Worksheet C1, Column 2, 3, 4, or 5 is . . .	② What makes this emotion difficult for me is . . .	③ In the past or in the future, AddictBrain may use this emotion in the following way . . .
Grief	I have difficulty with grief and would use to avoid it. It seems like it is always there right under the surface.	AddictBrain keeps my grief about my son's death alive. It knows I hate to feel this way. My son would want me to feel better. AddictBrain wants me to hurt so I continue to drink.

① An important emotion from Worksheet C1, Column 2, 3, 4, or 5 is . . .	② What makes this emotion difficult for me is . . .	③ In the past or in the future, AddictBrain may use this emotion in the following way . . .

Question 2: With the help of your peers and staff, come up with a list of ways you can uncouple these emotions from AddictBrain. List several ideas below:

_____

_____

_____

_____

_____

_____

_____

Worksheet C4: Stories from My Life

Each of us has had important emotional experiences in our lives. To help you understand your feelings and to assist others, write a few paragraphs about three important emotional events during your life. The moments could be hard times where you felt hurt, abandoned, or otherwise mistreated. Or they could be times when you felt loved, noticed, or proud. Any other emotional state is fine as well. It may be the most challenging to write about an event when you felt a strong mix of different emotions all at the same time. When you write down the events, describe your emotional response. Also try to have the story tell how you felt. Title the story only after you have completed writing out the events.

Story #1

The event occurs when I was _____ years old.

The following people were part of this event:

_____   _____
Name   Relationship

_____   _____
Name   Relationship

_____   _____
Name   Relationship

_____   _____
Name   Relationship

This is what happened: _____

_____

_____

_____

_____

_____

_____

_____

I call this story: _____

At this very moment when writing about this event, I feel: _____

_____

_____

Story #2

The event occurs when I was ____ years old.

The following people were part of this event:

_____   _____
Name   Relationship

_____   _____
Name   Relationship

_____   _____
Name   Relationship

_____   _____
Name   Relationship

This is what happened: _____

_____

_____

_____

_____

_____

_____

_____

I call this story: _____

At this very moment when writing about this event, I feel: _____

_____

_____

Story #3

The event occurs when I was _____ years old.

The following people were part of this event:

_____   _____
Name   Relationship

_____   _____
Name   Relationship

_____   _____
Name   Relationship

_____   _____
Name   Relationship

This is what happened: _____

_____

_____

_____

_____

_____

_____

_____

_____

I will call this story: _____

At this very moment when writing about this event, I feel: _____

_____

_____

Domain C: Progress Assessment Form

Emotional Resilience—RecoveryMind Training

Domain C Recovery Skill	Date:						Date:						Date:					
	Patient			Staff			Patient			Staff			Patient			Staff		
	B	I	C	B	I	C	B	I	C	B	I	C	B	I	C	B	I	C
Is able to accurately identify feeling states in self.																		
Is able to identify accurately feeling states in others.																		
Can experience strong emotions without acting out or "acting in."																		
Has completed the **Emotions Acceptance Assignment** and has used it to look beneath default emotional reactions.																		
Recognizes the specific emotions or memories that AddictBrain commonly uses to induce relapse and has a written plan for each.																		
Recognizes specific feelings that were captured and felt only through addiction.																		
Recalls past traumatic or painful events and discloses the full range of emotions about these events.																		
If a mood disorder or other psychiatric or psychological condition is present, can articulate and understands how AddictBrain uses this condition to its own ends.																		
Recognizes how addiction has changed the experience of pleasure and joy, turning it into the empty pursuit of euphoria.																		
Has experienced pleasure without engaging in addiction.																		

This evaluation is completed by both the patient or client (self-assessment) and his or her therapist or staff members on this one form. After starting work on a skill, place the approximate start date in the column provided. The patient or client fills out the form first. A therapist or staff member performs the same evaluation, placing a check mark in each row that indicates progress in assigned Recovery Skills. This process may need to be repeated for a several times as work progresses in each domain.

A check mark in the **B** column signifies that work has begun. The **I** column should be checked if the patient is in an intermediate or midway through his or her work on this item, and the **C** column should be checked if the patient has made sufficient progress in the skill to move forward to his or her next task. Review and discussion of this form helps patients and therapists set clear treatment expectations and recovery goals.

Domain C: Emotional Awareness and Resilience Notes

1. C. Darwin. "The Expression of Emotions in Man and Animals." 370: Filiquarian, 2007.

2. P. Ekman, and W. V. Friesen. "Constants across Cultures in the Face and Emotion." *J Pers Soc Psychol* 17, no. 2 (1971): 124–29.

3. J. A. Russell. "Is There Universal Recognition of Emotion from Facial Expression? A Review of the Cross-Cultural Studies." *Psychol Bull* 115, no. 1 (1994): 102–41.

4. R. Adolphs. "Recognizing Emotion from Facial Expressions: Psychological and Neurological Mechanisms." *Behav Cogn Neurosci Rev* 1, no. 1 (2002): 21–62.

5. D. A. Havas, A. M. Glenberg, K. A. Gutowski, M. J. Lucarelli, and R. J. Davidson. "Cosmetic Use of Botulinum Toxin-a Affects Processing of Emotional Language." *Psychol Sci* 21, no. 7 (2010): 895–900.

6. R. Plutchik. "The Nature of Emotions." *American Scientist* 89, no. 4 (2001): 344–50.

7. S. L. Koole. "The Psychology of Emotion Regulation: An Integrative Review. " *Cognition and Emotion* 23, no. 1 (2008): 4-41.

8. F. A. Thorberg, R. M. Young, K. A. Sullivan, and M. Lyvers. "Alexithymia and Alcohol Use Disorders: A Critical Review." *Addict Behav* 34, no. 3 (2009): 237–45.

9. A. Marlatt, and D. Donovan. *Relapse Prevention, Maintenance Strategies in the Treatment of Addictive Behaviors.* Second ed.: Guilford Press, 2007.

10. G. Marlatt. "Surfing the Urge." Inquiring Mind, https://www.inquiringmind.com/article/2602_w_marlatt-interview-with-g-alan-marlatt-surfing-the-urge/.

11. S. Bowen, N. Chawla, and G. Marlatt. *Mindfulness-Based Relapse Prevention for Addictive Behaviors: A Clinician's Guide.* Guilford Press, 2010.

12. S. Bowen, K. Witkiewitz, S. L. Clifasefi, J. Grow, N. Chawla, S. H. Hsu, H. A. Carroll, *et al.* "Relative Efficacy of Mindfulness-Based Relapse Prevention, Standard Relapse Prevention, and Treatment as Usual for Substance Use Disorders: A Randomized Clinical Trial. " *JAMA Psychiatry* (2014).

13. A. Blatner. *Acting-In: Practical Applications of Psychodramatic Methods.* Third ed.: Springer Publishing Company, 1996.

Domain D: Internal Narrative
Skills Groups, Assignments, Worksheets, and the Progress Assessment Form

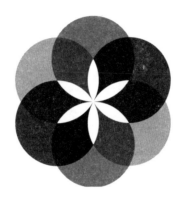

Chapter Overview

Work in Domain D focuses on rearranging thought patterns, points of view, and the narration of day-to-day reality that are counterproductive to a solid recovery. Our internal narrative has two components: the moment-to-moment internal statements we make that alter our ongoing mood and actions and the longer-term life stories that solidify self-concept. Both types of narrative are altered by AddictBrain. In Domain D, the focus is on thematic issues, how self-talk keeps the soil fertile for AddictBrain to grow and survive. Domain F, Relapse Prevention, addresses how short-term thoughts promote or dissuade relapse. The therapeutic approach for Domain D comes from many sources, among them are Cognitive Behavioral Therapy and Voice Therapy.[1]

Every one of us has "voices" in our heads; most experience them as thoughts, ideas, and a type of motivational pressure. They correct behavior, nag us to correct our actions, cajole us to improve, and tempt us to eat that dessert. The anthropologist Andrew Irving describes it in this manner:

> The capacity for a multifaceted, imaginative inner life encompassing internally represented speech, random urges, unfinished thoughts, inchoate imagery and much else besides—is an essential feature of the human condition and a principal means through which people understand themselves and others. Simply put, without people's inner expressions and imaginative lifeworlds there would be no social existence or understanding, at least not in a form we would recognize.[2]

Internal dialogue is inextricably linked with consciousness. It builds over our lifetime and has distinct qualities and repeated patterns by the time we reach adulthood. Our internal narrative is a critical part of the experience of being human. It defines who we are and how we relate to others in a social community.[3] Many schools of psychotherapy posit that parental constraint and control provide the foundation for internal narrative. During periods of self-discovery, we add our own voice to the mix. Our own adolescent narrative invariably emerges in direct conflict to previously internalized parental voices, (e.g., "It's important to try new things" countermands preexisting internalized parental phrases such as "Be careful, you might hurt yourself"). One central task of maturing into adulthood is to integrate these polar opposites and, in doing so, form a robust self-concept.

Addiction exploits our internal conflict. In the adolescent or young adult, alcohol or other drug use often is the reactive voice that, in a misguided attempt at self-definition, defies parental constraint and control. AddictBrain uses attempts at self-definition to foster alcohol and other drug use and attachment to addiction culture. This psychodynamic theme erupts to varying degrees in every addicted young adult. In many cases, the only emergent voices in an addicted adolescent's head are the constraining internalized voices of his parental figures and AddictBrain. This, I believe, accounts for much of the difficulty in treating this population.

Once one suffers from addiction, his or her internal narrative is deeply interlinked with shame. Those in the throes of an addiction illness "are strongly influenced or controlled by a destructive thought that first seduces the person into the addictive behavior and punishes them for indulging in it."[4] This invariably leads to self-castigation and shame, which in turn accelerates feelings of helplessness.

Some clients may label their critical inner voice as their conscience. The lay public describes addicts as people who "need more will power" and "lack a conscience." Literature and mythology equate our inner voice with our conscience (baby boomers recall Jiminy Cricket flying close to our ear, singing, "♫Always let your conscience be your guide♫"). One important task in Domain D, borrowed from Voice Therapy, is learning that this inner voice is not a conscience or a moral guide. What most distinguishes the inner voice from a conscience is its degrading, punishing quality. Its demeaning tone tends to increase our feelings of self-hatred, instead of motivating us to change undesirable actions in a constructive manner.[5, 1]

Therapists walk a tightrope here, attempting to increase self-insight without exacerbating self-hate. The journey here involves realizing hard truths; and addicts who are on the road to recovery are prone to shame, flogging themselves with the self-truths gained here. When working with patients in Domain D, the therapist must closely monitor their countertransference, lest it unconsciously align with the harsh self-talk of the client. Most patients will begin by alternating between AddictBrain and past shame-driven internal controls. The eventual goal is different, finding an internal voice that promotes self-care without harsh decree and continual recrimination. This goal is reflected in twelve-step support groups; here a nonjudgmental mutual supportive network supports abstinence and personal growth, combining it with unconditional acceptance and love.

Individuals who suffer from addiction begin treatment minimizing their illness, even when it is fulminant. As they improve, the client begins to say, "I was (or am) sicker than I thought." As insight accelerates, he or she may even argue with his or her peers about "who is sicker," asking staff to resolve a friendly argument about which patient wins the prize for the unhealthiest thinking. It is obviously best to avoid refereeing such disagreements. However, I have found this transition to be a good prognostic sign that appears when the bulk of denial falls. The astute therapist will notice one of the many paradoxes in addiction treatment: As individuals move from being sick to acquiring mental and emotional health, they identify with being sicker and sicker, certainly in their past but even in early recovery.

Pathological Euphemisms

The first task in Domain D is exploring how AddictBrain uses simple phrases to minimize addiction. Each patient will do this with different phraseology. Some might say, "I just took a nip to relax at the end of a day." A patient may say, "I borrowed my mother's hydrocodone." Healthcare professionals will "divert medications" rather than "steal drugs." All pill addicts use euphemistic terms for drugs, such as "my medication," "my pills," or "my helpers." (Note how the word "my" is spoken with affection and possessiveness). The list of language distortions is voluminous and proportional to the height of a patient's intellect and the depths of his or her defenses. Such subtle distortions of reality prevent insight; discovering and removing them stabilize self-perception.

I should spend a minute here discussing why the terms *addict* and *alcoholic* are not necessarily negative and counterproductive to use. These terms often carry pejorative connotations when uttered by the public. However, if we use lesser terms, we run the risk of trivializing this deadly disease and subtly colluding with our patient's unconscious hunger to hide behind a wall of normalcy. Although this manual uses terms like *individual with a substance use disorder* here, do not discourage patients from using alcoholic or addict if they find one of these fits best and helps them remember the severity of their illness.

Each patient arrives in treatment with a list of wordplays designed to "soften the blow," to push the nightmare away. The therapist's job is to help the patient identify these turns of a phrase that keep him or her sick. Never pass up a moment to query patients when they use euphemisms that are deeply contorted. When taking an intake history, a patient might use a euphemism for a life-altering medical event, such as " . . . and there was the time I went to the hospital because I fell." Feigning confusion between events, you could ask, "Is this the time you were on a ladder painting your house and fell, fracturing your leg and arm and suffering a traumatic brain injury?" The skill here is encouraging curiosity without a trace of hostility. Concept clarification and curiosity, rather than reproach, open the door to self-examination.

AddictBrain is predictable. If the illness returns, these very same twists of language predictably reappear. After going through the exercises in Domain D, the return of pathological euphemisms used by the individual indicates not only to the individual, but hopefully to his or her physician or therapist, that their illness is returning. When shared with family members, friends, and an AA/NA sponsor, the patient's network can pick up disease regression should it occur, often months before substance use or addiction relapse actually occurs.

A Deeper Appreciation of Denial

In Domain B, patients were introduced to the basics of denial. Here, it will be explored more fully. *Denial* has become a catchall term for distorted addictive thinking. Staff may use it so often and so incorrectly, that patients become confused saying, "I know you think I am in denial, but I think I am ready to go to that family function." In a related movement, addiction treatment has been urged to be more positivist and empowering of our patients. These two factors have given the concept of denial an undeserved bad rap. Our minds are by nature discriminating engines. We must know where we **are** before we can set a course to where we are **going**. Therefore, RecoveryMind Training retains the term denial and refines its use to specific defense mechanisms.

In an effort to develop a deeper understanding of defense mechanisms, I encourage everyone to read Vaillant's masterpiece, *Adaptation to Life*[6], published in 1977. In its original analytic meaning, denial is literally a "denial of external reality." In denying external reality, the individual has rearranged his or her perception of the external world. This is different from other defense mechanisms and more restrictive than the offhand lingo used in addiction treatment. When using repression, for example, someone experiences a change in her internal world (e.g., "Even after he said all that to me, I really am not angry"). Addiction therapists have unfortunately lumped together all defense mechanisms under the term denial. It is much more valuable to see this as one of the many defenses addicts exhibit. In RecoveryMind Training, I define any maneuver AddictBrain employs to keep its hapless victim from acting in the service of recovery as a defense mechanism and is therefore one part of the "Denial Complex." Many of these elements are simply defense mechanisms that everyone employs from time to time to manage disquieting affect—we all employ them from time to time. They could simply be called "addiction defense mechanisms." In a nod to the preexisting term that has been floating around addiction care for decades, I have chosen to refer to them as the "Denial Complex."

Let's look at each of the elements of the Denial Complex. They are:
- **Rationalization:** "I deserve a drink after my terrible day at work." Or, "I know I have many DWI/DUIs, but I am a good driver, I am a better driver drunk than most people are sober!"
- **Minimization:** "I only had three beers before the accident. And the accident was not that bad." (Reality: totaled car with two other people in the car while blindly intoxicated.)

- **Blaming**: "My husband is so controlling he makes me drink" and "My doctor is at fault because she prescribed the medications." (Reality: patient "doctor shops" going to three or four doctors to obtain pills.)

- **Going vague**: "I started drinking in college, but it was not that much, only when friends had alcohol." When asked how it progressed, the patient responds, "You know I drink now and then, sometimes more and sometimes less." As the Denial Complex improves, his or her use history improves dramatically. I say, "Vagueness is the friend of AddictBrain; clarity is the friend of RecoveryMind."

- **Intellectualization**: "You say I have a drug problem. Tell me again about which parts of my brain are causing this to happen. I want to understand this better."

- **Projection**: "You have the wrong person in treatment. You should see my wife (or husband) drink. They are the person who really has a problem."

- **Hostility as defense**: "Why are you asking all these questions?" or "You are just trying to tell me what is the right and wrong way to live!"

- **Dishonesty** or **Lying**: Although lying (dishonesty, stretching the truth, manipulating events, shading the truth, scamming, and so forth) is not commonly labeled a defense mechanism, it is included here. Addiction is one great big lie. Even when brain functioning is compromised in other areas, in individuals with addiction retain the ability for subterfuge. Lying starts out as a way of covering one's tracks and becomes increasingly automatic, moving from conscious manipulation to automatic reaction. Chapter Five of the AA Big Book, in discussing those who may not be able to recover, states, "They are naturally incapable of grasping and developing a manner of living which demands rigorous honesty."[7] Honesty is critical for recovery, and in most cases, dishonesty is a natural manifestation of AddictBrain.

- And finally, **Denial**: "I can quit anytime I feel like it." "The incident my son told you about did not happen. I do not know why he makes up such things about me." People who have addiction use denial to avoid seeing medical complications: "I do not have any problems walking and do not need that wheelchair," (voiced when feebly shuffling about after multiple falls in the detoxification unit).

The central tenet of work in this area is that the more patients understand the mechanisms of the Denial Complex, the faster they spot and correct their self-defeating distortions.

Patients recognize elements of the Denial Complex in others first. Most treatment centers have traditionally used this technique to promote community wellness. Patients who are further along can accelerate their own recovery by gently pointing out defense mechanisms in others. If done with compassion, it helps all community members. If a patient becomes agitated when one of his fellows "isn't getting" proper insightful feedback, it either indicates residual defenses or self-hostile feelings about previous blindness—which are explored as the group process evolves. In group therapy, we say, "You spot it, you got it."

In RecoveryMind Training, all the conventional group techniques are used to scrape away pathological AddictBrain defenses. The one twist that speeds this process comes from granular instruction regarding elements in the Denial Complex. Defenses are normalized; they become a normal part of life. However, they are also signposts that direct the therapist's attention to therapeutic work that increases insights and ensures a solid recovery.

Domain D includes two denial worksheets (The Denial Rating Scale–D2 and The Mechanics of Denial–D3) and one denial-related worksheet (The Inner Voice of AddictBrain–D4), assignment and two Skills Groups focused on helping patients recognize defense mechanisms in self and others. This manual provides many tools to manage the pernicious problem of denial. Obviously, every patient will not be assigned or complete every worksheet.

Part of the team's job in Domain D is to consider which of the denial worksheets will best work with a given patient. The Denial Rating Scale, Worksheet D2 is helpful for patients who cannot grasp where they are in the process of change, patients who see denial as a light switch (either "in denial" or "completely self-aware"). It is also helpful for individuals who have difficulty envisioning the process of change. Worksheet D2 is the most frequently used product in this regard. Worksheet D3–The Mechanics of Denial is best suited for individuals who have the psychological insight needed to parse through denial mechanisms. It is most commonly assigned to patients with one or more "sticky" defense mechanisms and who would benefit from this worksheet. Patients with unconscious but recalcitrant blaming defenses, for example, would benefit from completing this assignment and, even more importantly, reviewing it during Assignment Group. Patients with especially cruel or destructive internal dialogue are good candidates for Worksheet D4–The Inner Voice of AddictBrain. When such patients review Worksheet D4 in Assignment Group therapy, they begin the process of unwinding such interior dialogue.

It is important to note that work in this area also helps remove barriers to interpersonal effectiveness, improve mood, and increase insight in general. Defense styles are sticky, even after considerable time in recovery; a client will continue to use his preferred defense style in dealing with life issues. Therefore, a thorough examination of an individual's favored defensive types will help sustain recovery and increase his satisfaction with day-to-day interactions with others. Decreasing hostile interior dialogue substantively improves depression; decreasing self-talk is one of the central tasks in cognitive behavioral therapy. Thus, work in Domain D is especially important for patients with comorbid psychiatric disorders. Note that therapeutic work in Domain D is placed before work in Domain E. One must quiet the derogatory, self-directed internal hostility to some degree before satisfactory connection with others can occur.

The goals in Domain D are the following:
- Learning to recognize and correct pathological euphemisms, language that protects AddictBrain thinking.
- Identifying one's own favorite defense mechanisms and correcting their distortions.
- Recognizing AddictBrain's inner voice and taking corrective action to prevent unconscious reaction to that inner dialogue.
- Correlating addiction internal dialogue with other past coping mechanisms and negative self-talk.

There are three Skills Groups in Domain D:
D1) Identifying and correcting pathological euphemisms
D2) Role-playing the Denial Complex
D3) The internal voice of AddictBrain

There are four Assignment Group tasks in Domain D:
D1) Euphemisms for Additive Behaviors
D2) The Denial Rating Scale
D3) The Mechanics of Denial (Denial Complex)
D4) The Inner Voice of AddictBrain

There are five Worksheets and corresponding Assignment Group Tasks in Domain D:
D1) The **Pathological Euphemisms** Worksheet
D2) **The Denial Rating Scale** Worksheet
D3) **The Mechanics of Denial** Worksheet
D4) The **Inner Voice of AddictBrain** Worksheet
D5) The **List of Dishonesties** Worksheet

Domain D: Skills Groups

Skills Group D1: Pathological Euphemisms

Skills Group D1 is a simple and raucous group. The leader begins the group by labeling it as a brainstorming session. In brainstorming, there are no right or wrong answers. Members of the group are encouraged to disclose the sad, silly, and absurd ways they use language to "make light of," minimize, or distort using behaviors. Sometimes it is helpful to have a large whiteboard with one group member writing down the group's responses. A marijuana user may shout out, "I called it my smoky time." The leader suggests categories if the members are stuck. Suggested categories are:

- What you call your drugs or alcohol
- What you call your hiding places
- What you call your using locations
- What you call the negative consequences of using
- The euphemisms you use to describe:
    - Family discord
    - Medical complications
    - Psychological consequences

If there is time left at the end of the brainstorming session, the leader asks the group members to describe particularly surprising euphemisms realized during the session. The leader may also ask which euphemism was particularly dark or evil. This Skills Group prepares individuals for Worksheet D1.

Skills Group D2: The Denial Complex

Skills Group D2 is a role-playing group. The group starts by encouraging members to disclose a thought, saying, or interpersonal defense that is part of their denial. Several members may participate. The leader carefully listens for a particular scenario that can be effectively expanded into a role-play. For example, one member might state, "I always told myself I drank to get away from my husband who was so controlling." The leader invites this individual to participate in a role-play session. The identified protagonist stands up along with the group leader and establishes the stage. The protagonist enrolls her controlling husband if she can tolerate the resultant distress. Once enrolled, the protagonist trains the enrolled "husband" actor in what to say. The husband-actor verbalizes back to the protagonist and the leader ensures this feels historically accurate. Then, the leader suggests that they bring out the voice of her denial. Once enrolled, this voice may say something like, "The only way you can tolerate this is if you have a drink." Or "This is so oppressive; the only way to get away is to just get drunk." As with all role-play, it is critical that the leader ask a patient for a clear wording of her thoughts, refining and sharpening the dialogue, and then feeding that back to the actor for refinement and review.

At this point, often the scene is stopped briefly. Other group members are asked to identify the denial mechanism that is at play in the current scene. The leader then announces a reactivation of the role-play. If appropriate and if it feels genuine and correct to the protagonist, the leader suggests enrolling a protective voice or a voice of recovery, or both. The voice of recovery might say, "If you drink to get away from your husband, you lose twice. Once because you do not get away, twice because your AddictBrain is even more controlling." This Skills Group clarifies defenses through externalization and opens the door to alternative understanding and behaviors.

The scene is disenrolled and all actors return to their seats. Sharing is encouraged. If another group member begins a critique of the previous role-play, the leader stops this abruptly. Group members may share their own nuances of this defense mechanism and the scene, helping every group member understand his or her own version of the Denial Complex.

Skills Group D3: The Internal Voice of AddictBrain

Skills Group D3 is in many ways similar to Skills Group D2. They often begin in a very similar manner. One actor-auxiliary always enrolled in this role-play is the voice of AddictBrain. The leader carefully and surgically refines the AddictBrain voice watching the facial features and body language of the protagonist as they listen to AddictBrain's words. The leader ensures the words uttered by AddictBrain are accurate in meaning and tone. The leader responding to this defeat may say, "This is what it has been like for you, isn't it?"

If effective, the protagonist looks up at the leader her countenance asking for help and direction. At this point, the leader has two choices: Either lead the protagonist into a deeper family of origin scene (which was most likely the genesis of the Inner Voice) or offer an alternative for the protagonist's here-and-now situation. Stronger and more inquisitive patients will want to delve into their past. If the leader has the experiential therapy skills, a brief scene regarding the patient's family of origin ensues. If not, the leader may suggest a "what if" scenario based in the present or future.

This role-play commonly introduces the "Voice of Recovery." The leader carefully constructs this voice with a phrase such as "I know it may be hard to image, but consider for a moment what might have happened if you heard a recovery voice. It might say . . ." Once enrolled, the Voice of Recovery would suggest alternatives to the protagonist. If possible, the protagonist suggests these alternatives. The alternatives are clarified and fed back to the protagonist through this actor. Many phrases are repeated looking for just the right supportive tone. The leader may ask, "If you felt the drive to use right now, what do you need to hear to break away from this urge?"

Once the scene feels complete, all actors disenroll and return to their seats. Other patients share their experience. They may describe how their voice would have sounded to them. Once again, criticism is strongly discouraged.

Domain D: Assignment Groups Tasks

Remember that in Domain D, patients may be assigned one or more of the Domain D Worksheets. When a worksheet is assigned, it is expected that patients bid for time in Assignment Group to review his or her worksheet with his or her therapist or peers.

Assignment Group Task D1: Pathological Euphemisms

In this Assignment Group, the protagonist reads his or her list of euphemisms. He or she reads the euphemism first, providing a context in which the euphemism has occurred in the past. "My first euphemism is 'get adjusted.' I would use this euphemism at the end of a workday where I felt out of sorts. I would say to my drinking friends, 'I am out of whack. I need to **get adjusted**. Anyone want to join me?'" The protagonist would then state a more accurate phrase for this euphemism, "This was code for simply going to our bar and getting drunk or at least really high." Finally, the protagonist describes what AddictBrain got out of this euphemism, "I was able to blame my drinking on my job and to view my drinking as a repair for a problem rather than a worse problem than my work."

Other patients provide feedback from their list and relating to euphemisms that remind them of their own distorted phrases. At the end of the list, the therapist invites the group members to suggest other unmentioned pathological euphemisms that the protagonist has used in their presence while in treatment. These are then added to the worksheet, and the protagonist is instructed to fill out responses to group-identified items as additional homework.

Assignment Group Task D2: The Denial Rating Scale

If a patient has been assigned the Denial Rating Scale (DRS) Worksheet, he or she begins this task stating his or her current score on the DRS. Using the descriptions of each DRS level the protagonist justifies his score. Other patients ask questions and gently correct distortions about a patient's self-perception. If the leader sees the protagonist has a realistic understanding of his current DRS, he proceeds by reading his scores over the past several weeks. Again, other patients ask questions and provide feedback about how they see the protagonist's denial rating.

Staff members need to consistently correct judgments about one score or another during this exercise. Competitive patients may take this opportunity to set up hierarchical relationships within the group. This must be strongly discouraged for honest self-appraisal.

Assignment Group Task D3: The Denial Complex

After the protagonist has bid for time, he or she reads the Denial Complex phrases from Worksheet D3. After each item, a discussion of the denial mechanism ensues. During this Assignment Group task, it is helpful if all group members have a list of the elements of the Denial Complex at hand to refer to for quick reference. The group discusses the subtleties and difficulties in understanding each of the denial mechanisms, facilitated by the leader. It is important for the leader to reiterate that differentiating the different defense mechanisms is often difficult. Some patients may never be able to do this completely. However, it has been observed that when a patient uses an element of the Denial Complex frequently, he or she has difficulty understanding or identifying it in others.

Group members who have not completed Worksheet D4 find this Assignment Group helpful. Limited self-disclosure by non-protagonist members is encouraged.

Assignment Group Task D4: The Inner Voice of AddictBrain

In this group task, the protagonist reads Worksheet D4. As is explained elsewhere, this worksheet is best reserved for individuals who need to connect AddictBrain with premorbid negative or destructive self-talk (usually hostile introjects that resulted from childhood situations). The purpose of the worksheet and thus this Assignment Group Task is different from Assignment D3. In D3, the goal is to help a patient understand the nuances of his or her denial and thus gain enlightenment about his or her addiction. In contrast, task D4 helps a patient understand how his or her long-standing negative or self-destructive self-talk has been hijacked by AddictBrain worsening addiction and degrading his or her self-concept.

The protagonist reads the list, stating what AddictBrain says to him or her and relating that to other internal dialogue related to other issues. For example, a patient's AddictBrain may say, "You should drink so other people at the party will enjoy your company." The related inner voice may be "People don't like you much, but you are a little more fun when you're high."

Domain D: Internal Narrative Worksheets

Overview of Worksheets

The power of worksheets in Domain D comes from understanding internal processes, removing them from the head, and exposing them to the light of day. When completing a written assignment, patients develop distance as they write their thoughts or beliefs down on paper. This is amplified when they are reviewed, first personally and then in the Assignment Group. Saying some of the negative, patently absurd thoughts in our head out loud produces some correction of false beliefs. Working them through carefully in Assignment Group or even Skills Group creates shifts in understanding that are light years ahead of "sitting in the corner and thinking about it."

These assignments also help correct some of the distortions produced by depressive illnesses, anxiety disorders, and characterological issues. The Cognitive Behavioral Therapy provided by these worksheets and group therapy setting is powerful and healing.

As described above, patients may be assigned any or all of these worksheets. The decisions about which worksheet to use comes from multiple sources including: the words a patient uses, how superficial or deep his or her understanding of denial as a process may be, his or her level of psychological insight, the number of previous treatments and relapses, and the therapist's insight into the client's self-hostility from his or her internal dialogue.

There are five worksheets in Domain D:

D1) The **Pathological Euphemisms** Worksheet. In this worksheet, the client records simple phrases and thoughts that minimize his or her addiction through euphemisms. This worksheet is based upon the RecoveryMind Training principle that subtle changes in language can distort or clarify understanding. Every addicted individual develops a series of euphemisms that minimize, deny, or rationalize addictive behaviors. RecoveryMind Training, through the use of "re-languaging," corrects these subtle but pervasive distortions.

D2) The **Denial Rating Scale**. This worksheet is a staff and patient completed subjective scale that ranks the severity of denial. The Denial Rating Scale was developed many years ago by Dr. Jeff Goldsmith and his colleagues. The patient reads the description and places him- or herself on an eight-point scale. Dispassionate assessment will help patients (and staff) accept denial as normal. It resolves at different rates in different people. If assigned this worksheet, the patient scores him- or herself daily. During Assignment Group, the patient reports and receives corrective feedback as to his or her denial level at that moment. This deepens understanding about this elusive concept, helps the patient recognize day-to-day fluctuation, and maps a clear path for the recovery journey.

D3) **The Mechanics of Denial** Worksheet. This worksheet prods the patient to record an exhaustive list of defenses that block acceptance of his or her addiction disorder. This worksheet expands curiosity about defense mechanisms by categorizing them using a simple schema. While completing this worksheet the client asks his or her family, peers in treatment, and staff to help catalog his or her Denial Complex. This worksheet may be reviewed in Assignment Group if the therapist feels it would help solidify learning.

D4) The **Inner Voice of AddictBrain** Worksheet. In this worksheet, patients detail the "inner voice" or "internal dialogue" manufactured by AddictBrain. This worksheet is like D3 above but focuses more on a patient's internal process and less on interpersonal interaction. Refer to the Assignment Group task associated with this worksheet for more information.

D5) The **List of Dishonesties** Worksheet. This worksheet is assigned to an individual who has a complex web of dishonesties that enshroud his or her addiction and block progress in recovery. Using a less pejorative word than dishonesties (e.g., dissimulation) has been considered, but the most direct word seems to work best. When assigning this worksheet, be careful not to imply that a given individual is simply "a liar." Coach all patients that dishonesty is part of addiction. Most often, there is no Assignment Group task for this worksheet since it promotes judgmentalism and invites group hostility. That said, some clients will have the ego strength to review this list in group, but this should be done selectively and with caution.

Worksheet D1: Pathological Euphemisms

Everyone who suffers from addiction has hidden his or her sickness from him- or herself. One of the most powerful ways this occurs is through subtle distortions of language. Some of these are amusing, created by the industry that caters to us—in my hometown there is a bar named "The Office." The individual with alcohol use disorder can grin to himself while stating to a coworker or friend, "I have to go to the office."

Merriam-Webster defines a *euphemism* as "a mild or pleasant word or phrase that is used instead of one that is unpleasant or offensive." AddictBrain, acting like a smooth salesman, twists words or phrases that accurately describe one's addiction and its related behaviors. In doing so, it keeps the individual from seeing the problem for what it is. These euphemisms are dangerous; they hide the truth and keep those with addiction unaware. We therefore call them pathological—they keep the individual sick.

Question 1: Below is a table where you will place your rationalizations, word phrases, and other euphemisms that hid the truth about your addiction. The list is divided into several categories. Several examples appear at the beginning of each category, to help you get started. Overwrite or edit the examples with your own words that minimized your addiction and go on to fill out as many of your rationalizations as possible in column ②. Expand the shorter phrase to a more complete meaning in column ③. Then enter what the euphemism was attempting to hide about your addiction in column ④. Place a check mark in column ① if you used this type of euphemism often.

① ✓	② Pathological Euphemism	③ How I said it to myself or when I said it was . . .	④ The truth I was trying to hide from others and myself was . . .
Obtaining Drugs or Alcohol			
	I "diverted" or "obtained" drugs		I was stealing drugs.
	I store alcohol or drugs in "convenient" places		I made sure I would not run out.
	I went to the doctor.		I scammed doctors for drugs.
	I went to see my friend.		Going to a dangerous place to meet a guy who was not a friend, just a dealer.
	They don't need them		Spoken when stealing drugs from others (medicine cabinet, etc.).

① ✓	② **Pathological Euphemism**	③ **How I said it to myself or when I said it was . . .**	④ **The truth I was trying to hide from others and myself was . . .**
Using Chemicals			
	My little reward		*Using drugs or alcohol*
	I just had a nip, took a taste, tried a little, or said yes to a little drink.		*I drank because I always did so, even if it did not help me feel better.*
	I drank to calm my nerves or to help me be more social.		*I drank because I always did so, even if it did not help.*
Emotional Consequences			

① ✓	② Pathological Euphemism	③ How I said it to myself or when I said it was . . .	④ The truth I was trying to hide from others and myself was . . .
	Drinking (or drug use) is the only thing that makes me feel better.		Although I do not want to see it, I wind up feeling worse about myself.
	Using calms my nerves.		The anti-anxiety effects of drugs or alcohol has stopped working.
	I need to relax		I cannot relax without using.
Physical Consequences			
	My liver can take it.		The amount I drink is damaging my liver.
	I have a strong constitution.		I am using enough to cause problems.
	My doctor told me I have essential tremor.		Alcohol or drug induced tremors.

① ✓	② **Pathological Euphemism**	③ **How I said it to myself or when I said it was . . .**	④ **The truth I was trying to hide from others and myself was . . .**
Legal Consequences			
	The police were out to get me.		*I was driving while intoxicated.*
	I was not a drug dealer.		*I had financial problems and had to sell to make ends meet.*
Relationship Consequences			

① ✓	② **Pathological Euphemism**	③ **How I said it to myself or when I said it was . . .**	④ **The truth I was trying to hide from others and myself was . . .**
	My wife (husband, children, parents, S.O.) make me drink		*Loved ones are irritated by my using*
	I drink / drug to tolerate my husband / wife / S.O.		*My using is only making troubled relationships worse*
Damage to Others			
	They brought this on themselves		*I was hurtful to someone and justified my actions while using.*

① ✓	② Pathological Euphemism	③ How I said it to myself or when I said it was . . .	④ The truth I was trying to hide from others and myself was . . .
Other			

Worksheet D2: The Denial Rating Scale

One of the most difficult and pernicious aspects of addiction is how it hides itself from its victims. AddictBrain spends an enormous amount of your brain energy cloaking itself inside your mind. This is one of the reasons why individuals have more energy for other life goals when they enter recovery. Once in recovery, AddictBrain no longer saps your mental energy to remain hidden. Denial is normal and resolves at different rates in every person with a substance use disorder. One way of helping it recede is to understand it better. When you are curious (rather than self-hostile) about your denial you shine the light of day upon it and, in doing so, it fades faster. Denial is not like a light switch. You do not have it one day and it is gone the next. AddictBrain uses myriad defenses to keep you from taking firm action to get better.

If you were assigned this exercise, you may be saying to yourself, "Wait a minute, I already worked on my denial in Domain B! I completed a First Step already. Why am I doing this now?" The reason is simple. Eliminating denial is not a single event; it is a process. Now that you are further along in your recovery, you are more able to see the subtle qualities of AddictBrain, how it carefully and quietly undoes your hard-earned insight, how pockets of denial still plague your recovery. This worksheet takes a deeper dive into denial.

To further your work, there is a powerful tool called the Denial Rating Scale (DRS). Dr. Jeff Goldsmith developed this tool many years ago. It allows you, your therapist, and others to evaluate denial using a simple eight-point scale. When assigned this worksheet, you will reexamine your level of denial at assigned intervals. It is best to repeat this quick assessment during your morning or evening reflection. You may be assigned this daily for two weeks (Question 1), weekly for three months (Question 2), or both. If you work on this worksheet faithfully, you will most likely find that your denial waxes and wanes over time. This is completely normal. Try to be analytical and dispassionate in your self-appraisal; above all else, try not to judge your responses as good or bad/right or wrong.

Question 1 (Two-Week Evaluation Period): Before you begin this exercise, place the start date in Column ⓪ of Week 1. Then ignore the days of the week in Week 1 before today.

Next, read through the description of the Denial Rating Scale at the end of this worksheet, looking for the value that best describes your current thoughts and beliefs (not what you are telling others!). Be objective, stand outside of yourself for a moment, and evaluate your recent thoughts and actions. Start on the proper day of the week. Each day for two weeks, take a few minutes to review the denial rating scale while considering your status at the moment of the review. Enter the value in the correct day of the week. Note that this may go into Week 3 depending on which day of the week you begin this exercise.

My Denial Rating

	⓪ Start Date	① Sunday	② Monday	③ Tuesday	④ Wednesday	⑤ Thursday	⑥ Friday	⑦ Saturday
Week 1								
Week 2								
Week 3								

Question 2 (Three-Month Evaluation): Before beginning this exercise, select a day of the week where you will look back on the preceding week and evaluate your position on the denial rating scale. Many people pick a point at the end of the week (e.g., Friday or Sunday). Enter the day of the week you have chosen to self-evaluate here: _____. Write the start date of the first and subsequent two months in column 0 (zero) below. If you start in the middle of a month, enter your scale value in the appropriate week and begin the next month with the first week. If you start mid-month, you will go into a fourth calendar month to complete the three-month assignment. With this assessment I recommend you get feedback from your sponsor or peers in recovery.

During the next three months, on the day of the week you have chosen, review the Denial Rating Scale. Think back on the previous week to get an objective view of where your denial stands. Enter the number in the table below. The assignment is complete when you have entered a value each week for three months.

	Name of Month	⓪ Start Date	① Week 1	② Week 2	③ Week 3	④ Week 4
Month 1						
Month 2						
Month 3						
Month 4						

The Denial Rating Scale

Modified from the work of Jeffery Goldsmith, MD

Level 1: "No Problem"

If you are at this level, you tend to deny any emotional or family problems. You may be in treatment as a requirement of probation, family pressure, or other external factors. You may feel little or no commitment to change because nothing is wrong. You tend to be only marginally cooperative with treatment. You may be defensive or confused by the focus on alcohol or other drug issues. People at this level rarely bring up the issue of addiction spontaneously. You tend to see no reason to control alcohol or other drug use. You probably feel your use is easy to control and see your use as fun. You believe alcohol and other drugs are only affecting your family to the extent that your use upsets others. You may state you can choose or have chosen to refrain from drinking or other drug use (or quitting altogether) for various reasons. In either case treatment does not seem to have any value or you have nothing you feel you need to discuss.

Level 2: "A Problem"

If you are at this level, you do not think you have a problem with alcohol or other drugs. You may endorse other problems spontaneously such as anxiety ("nerves") or depression or problems with relationships, children, health, or money. When you are at this level you often feel misunderstood, your therapist or treatment staff seems to be focusing on the wrong problem or problems. As a result, you may feel out of step with other clients or patients or that you are in the wrong place. You may have some concern that drinking or drug use could become an issue in the future. People who score at this level tend to cooperate with treatment voluntarily, even if they "don't belong."

Level 3: "Addiction Is a Problem"

People at this level agree that alcohol or other drugs contribute to life difficulties. When you are in Level 3, however, you tend to believe your difficulties are controllable. Drinking or drug use is seen as a reaction to and a way of coping with, life stress. Gaining control over these difficulties will therefore control the drinking or drug use. You do not believe or accept that addiction is the primary problem. You find it hard to accept that you have an addiction disorder that is distinct from your other difficulties. You may not see your addictive difficulties as progressive. You are very skeptical about consistent loss of control. People at this level believe that someone who has a substance use disorder drinks more or uses more drugs than they do. You may often feel defensive when the staff focuses on what they believe are your addiction problems.

Level 4: "Sobriety May Help, but I Can Control It"

The person at this level accepts the idea of having a major problem with alcohol or other drugs and may even call him- or herself an alcoholic or a person with a substance use disorder. If you are at this level, however, you have a fairly strong conviction (which you may hold to yourself) that you can soon return to controlled drinking or drug use. People at this level who are not in formal treatment tend to try limiting their drinking or drug use. They may even be successful for short periods of time. They may ask others to "have just a sip" or to approve their attempts to control their use. Individuals at this level may report having a history of addiction in the past. If a person at this level stops drinking, he or she usually feels like a logical decision was made with little attached emotion or meaning. You may sense that your substance problem is erratic and perplexing but feel little or no urgency about your need to really stop.

Level 5: "Sobriety Will Help"

Someone at this level recognizes that his or her drinking or drug use is out of control and that life is out of control due to addiction. If you are at this level, you may feel conscious anxiety, guilt, or shame about your loss of control or addiction behaviors. If recently sober, your worry and anxiety may come from concerns about losing your family or job, winding up in jail or the hospital, or even going insane. People at this level are focused on how overwhelming their loss of control is, rather than what they should do about it. They accept the concept that their drinking is too much to control by themselves. They tend to turn to a therapist, sponsor, or meeting seeking control. They feel an internal commitment to change and can accept that addiction is an illness but have yet to understand the numerous implications of the work ahead.

Level 6: "Sobriety Is Easy"

The person at Level 6 has a solid commitment to sobriety. The anxiety of the previous level has sharply decreased. Some people at this level feel great. This phenomenon has been described as the "honeymoon" or "pink cloud" phase of recovery. This does not occur with everyone, however. Others feel miserable. The defining feature of this stage is a sense that recovery seems easier than previously thought. When at this stage, you may minimize the degree to which life has become entwined with alcohol or other drugs. Consequently, you will tend to underestimate the number of changes that must occur to stay sober and to rebuild your life (family, job, friends, and the like).

Level 7: "Sobriety Is Difficult"

An individual at this level experiences a return of anxiety, but this time the anxiety about broader issues such as reconstructing a whole life and making amends, saving a marriage, and the like. An individual at this level realizes his or her own role in repairing the past and seeks reassurance and support for the struggle, rather than asking others to change. Some individuals are less interested in exploring the past or present for deeper psychological meaning. Individuals at this level focus more on exercising control, problem-solving, social skills, and making amends.

Level 8: "Life Is Difficult"

Individuals at this level have gained confidence that life is possible and even quite pleasant without alcohol or other drugs. They appreciate some of the subtle dilemmas of existence and exhibit age-appropriate maturity. They bump up against and notice limitations of their personality style and often feel a desire to explore them. Level 8 is an excellent time to begin deeper self-exploration because the person with a substance use disorder has sufficient stability about his or her feelings, thoughts, and behaviors to work on these issues without relapse. Such a person accepts the self-image as someone with the chronic addiction condition. They know how easy it would be to fall back to drinking or drug use but are not threatened by this knowledge. People in Level 8 have most likely been sober a year or more.

Worksheet D3: The Mechanics of Denial

Everyone has heard the phrase "You're in denial." Most people with addiction disorders have heard it more than once. But what does this phrase mean? Denial is a complex process, driven by AddictBrain that keeps you from recognizing the negative consequences of your substance use or behavioral addiction. By keeping you in the dark, AddictBrain ensures that it can run effectively in stealth mode, constantly eroding your mental and physical health and destroying your self-esteem.

This worksheet is designed to help you understand the many aspects of this thing called "denial." If you are a bit confused about denial, you are not alone; the addiction treatment and recovery community has confused this concept over the years. Angry relatives, employers, friends, or even therapists may have thrown the word denial at you in anger, as if denial is a characteristic of stupidity or evil intent. Actually, denial is a natural part of the illness. For many, it is the most important stumbling block in early recovery.

Used in the world of addiction treatment, *denial* refers to many common psychological defenses. For clarity, RecoveryMind Training groups together all the AddictBrain defenses into a term: "Denial Complex." You will learn that denial itself is more accurately **one** of the defense mechanisms included in the Denial Complex. I believe exploring and properly labeling the ways AddictBrain hides is very important. Looking deeply and using precise language helps clear a path to sobriety.

The AddictBrain tricks that are part of the Denial Complex are:
- **Rationalization (R)**: "I deserve a drink after my terrible day at work." Or "I know I have many DWI/DUIs, but I am a good driver. I am a better driver drunk than most people are sober!"
- **Minimization (M)**: "I only had three beers before the accident. And the accident was not that bad." (Reality: totaled a car while driving with two other people while blindly intoxicated.)
- **Blaming (B)**: "My husband is so controlling he makes me drink." "My doctor is at fault because she prescribed the medications." (Reality: patient "doctor shops" going to three or four doctors to obtain pills.)
- **Going Vague (V)**: "I started drinking in college, but it was not that much, only when friends had alcohol." When asked how it progressed, your memory may seem remarkably cloudy, so you respond, "I drink now and then, sometimes more and sometimes less." As the Denial Complex improves, your recall of your using history will improve dramatically. I say, "Vagueness is the friend of AddictBrain; clarity is the friend of RecoveryMind."

- **Intellectualization (I)**: When faced with a painful or troubling aspect of your past, your mind distances from the emotion, moving into the intellect (e.g., "Tell me again about which parts of my brain are causing this to happen. I want to understand this better.")

- **Projection (P)**: Rather than accepting you're the behaviors and consequences of your addiction you displace them onto others. (e.g., "You have the wrong person in treatment. You should see my wife (or husband) drink. She (he) really has a drug problem.")

- **Hostility as Defense (H)**: When another patient or a therapist points out painful aspects of your addiction (when you feel shame), you get angry to keep from feeling guilt or shame. (e.g., "Why are you asking all these questions?!" or "You are just trying to tell me what is the right and wrong way to live. Who gives you that right?").

- **Dishonesty** or **Lying (L)**: Although lying (dishonesty, stretching the truth, manipulating events, shading the truth, scamming, and the like) is not commonly labeled a defense mechanism, it is included here. Individuals with addiction are effective at dissembling often, even when brain functioning is compromised in other areas. Lying starts out as a way of covering one's tracks and becomes increasingly automatic, moving from conscious manipulation to automatic reaction. Describing those who will not be able to attain recovery, Chapter 5 of the AA Big Book, states: "They are naturally incapable of grasping and developing a manner of living which demands rigorous honesty." Because honesty is critical for recovery and in most cases dishonesty has become a natural reflexive response, it is covered here.

- And of course, **Denial (D)**: "I can quit anytime I feel like it." "The incident my son told you about did not happen. I do not know why he makes up such things about me." You may also use denial to avoid seeing medical complications. "One time I ate bad oysters and became very sick. This is the reason for my elevated liver function tests. It is certainly not from drinking alcohol.").

After reading this list you may find yourself saying "This is complicated. I'm not a psychologist. Why do I have to learn all this stuff?" The answer is simple. The more you understand how your mind works, the easier it will be to correct unhelpful patterns of thinking. Most people who do not suffer from addiction do not need to understand defense mechanisms (although it certainly wouldn't hurt). Those with addiction illnesses, unfortunately, do not have this luxury. To effectively manage your illness, you need to understand yourself better than the average person.

To complete this worksheet, fill out common phrases you find yourself thinking or saying that promote relapse or continued use. Ask friends, relatives, or fellow patients to help you discover items you may not have recognized. Enter the phrase in column ①. Then, using the bulleted list above, go back and put an identifier in column ② that delineates the element of the Denial Complex you were using. If you are not sure which defense is at play with a given phrase, try your best. You and the therapist will review your list in Assignment Group and help with any items that are not clear.

① My denial would tell me (or I would say to others) . . .	② Denial Mechanism
I don't drink that much	M

① My denial would tell me (or I would say to others) . . .	② Denial Mechanism

Worksheet D4: The Inner Voice of AddictBrain

Each of us have different ways of seeing ourselves. One way we reinforce our self-image is through inner voices. All of us "talk to ourselves." We use our inner voice to keep us going ("You can do it!"). They can also keep us stuck ("You will never finish that project."). When we develop addiction, AddictBrain figures out how to use our strongest inner voices for its own purposes. If we frequently say to ourselves, "No matter how hard you try you eventually mess it up," AddictBrain twists this concept around and uses it to keep us from getting better ("You will work hard at this recovery thing but you will eventually relapse"). The stronger your inner voice is in any area, the more AddictBrain likes and uses it.

In this worksheet, you will examine the contents of your inner voice, searching for what AddictBrain has waylaid for its own use. To use this worksheet, start by thinking of phrases AddictBrain has always said to you (e.g., "Using is the only way I will feel better") and enter them in column ①. Then go back and try to relate this to past inner voices (e.g., "You are basically a depressive person and will always be that way"). If you can come up with a related inner voice or phrase put in in column ②. Don't worry if you cannot think of anything at the moment. Think about it and return later. If you are stumped, leave it blank.

Next, go through this exercise the other way. On a new line, enter a phrase that you have always said to yourself, an inner voice that pops up often. (e.g., "People never seem to get me, I always wind up feeling outside a group"). Enter this phrase in column ②. Then consider ways AddictBrain has used this inner voice for its own ends (e.g., "That feeling of being outside seems to slip away when you smoke a little weed or have a beer.") Put that AddictBrain voice in the same row in column ①.

When you have completed your list, go through it and rank the power of the AddictBrain or Inner Voice. By power, I mean how central it is to who you are and how strongly it has seemed to guide your self-concept over the years. Rate the power on a scale of 1 to 5 (1 being least strong, 5 being the strongest). Place that number in column ③ for each item in this worksheet.

You may have to spend time on this worksheet for a bit and then put it aside, returning to it when you have a sudden realization. This worksheet is hard for many people on many levels. Don't give up; it will strengthen your resilience to relapse.

① AddictBrain says to me . . .	② A related Inner Voice is . . .	③ Relative Power (1-5)

Worksheet D5: List of Dishonesties

Everyone tells fibs, uses white lies and, at times, is deceitful to others. People with substance use disorders are especially prone to dishonesty. Dishonesties start when the afflicted individual attempts to hide the painful truth from him- or herself. As many of you have discovered, this has led to a confusing mishmash of feelings and thoughts about your disease.

After a time, the dishonesties extend outside of the individual to others around him or her. Family members and loved ones are especially traumatized by dishonesty. In this worksheet, you will dig through the layers of dishonesties that feed AddictBrain. If you're assigned this worksheet, think hard and be thorough about your past dishonest behaviors. You will go through this exercise three times each time looking at dishonesties that are deeper and often more painful.

The first time through, right down lies you have told or tell others, but you personally knew were untrue. Put this in column ①. In column ②, write down how this lie protected your addiction. Then, in column ③ indicate whether the dishonesty was in the past (enter a **P**) or whether it is ongoing (enter an **O**). Try to recall as many of this type of dishonesty as possible.

The second time through, you should record lies you told or tell yourself alone but deep down know are untrue. Enter them as you did the first time through. The third and final time through, you will try to record past dishonesties that are so deep that you have not previously admitted the truth, even to yourself. This may prove difficult for some people. It is also the most painful type of dishonesty to reconcile. Take your time and return to this worksheet as necessary.

① The dishonesty is . . .	② It protects my addiction by . . .	③ Past or Ongoing?

① The dishonesty is . . .	② It protects my addiction by . . .	③ Past or Ongoing?

① The dishonesty is . . .	② It protects my addiction by . . .	③ Past or Ongoing?

Domain D: Progress Assessment Form

Internal Narrative: RecoveryMind Training

Domain D Recovery Skill	Date: Patient			Staff			Date: Patient			Staff			Date: Patient			Staff		
	B	I	C	B	I	C	B	I	C	B	I	C	B	I	C	B	I	C
Recognizes and corrects distortions of language (Pathological Euphemisms) that promote AddictBrain thinking.																		
Recognizes and correctly identifies elements of the Denial Complex in others.																		
Recognizes and correctly identifies elements of the Denial Complex in self.																		
Has identified the one or two of the elements of the Denial Complex he or she most often uses.																		
Has identified the one or two of the elements of the Denial Complex that cause family conflict.																		
Correctly identifies where he or she is on the Denial Rating Scale. Is able to note changes in DRS ratings from day to day.																		
Identifies self-defeating inner voices that have the potential to drive relapse.																		
Can connect these inner voices with self-concept and life messages that were internalized in childhood.																		
Has completed the List of Dishonesties Worksheet, if assigned, and is correcting this in daily interactions.																		

This evaluation is completed by both the patient or client (self-assessment) and his or her therapist or staff members on this one form. After starting work on a skill, place the approximate start date in the in the provided column. The patient or client fills out the form first. A therapist or staff member performs the same evaluation, placing a check mark in each row that indicates progress in assigned Recovery Skills. This process may need to be repeated for a several times as work progresses in each domain.

A check mark in the **B** column signifies that work has begun. The **I** column should be checked if the patient is in an intermediate or midway through his or her work on this item, and the **C** column should be checked if the patient has made sufficient progress in the skill to move forward to his or her next task. Review and discussion of this form helps patients and therapists set clear treatment expectations and recovery goals.

Domain D: Internal Narrative Notes

1. R. W. Firestone, and J. Catlett. "Voice Therapy." In *The Fantasy Bond: Structure of Psychological Defenses*, 298–321. New York, NY, US: Human Sciences Press, 1986.

2. A. Irving. "Strange Distance: Towards an Anthropology of Interior Dialogue." *Med Anthropol Quarterly* 25, no. 1 (2011): 22–44.

3. A. Irving. "Dangerous Substances and Visible Evidence: Tears, Blood, Alcohol, Pills." *Visual Studies* 25, no. 1 (2010): 24–35.

4. L. L. Firestone. "Breaking Free from Addiction." Glendon Association, http://www.psychalive.org/breaking-free-from-addiction/.

5. R. W. Firestone. *Voice Therapy: A Psychotherapeutic Approach to Self-Destructive Behavior*. Santa Barbara, CA: Glendon Association, 1988.

6. G. E. Vaillant. *Adaptation to Life*. First ed. Boston: Brown Little, 1977.

7. A. A. World Services. *Alcoholics Anonymous*. 4th ed. New York: A.A. World Services, 2013.

Domain E: Connectedness and Spirituality
Skills Groups, Assignments, Worksheets, and the Progress Assessment Form

Chapter Overview

Homo sapiens is a social and spiritual creature. Research suggests that social structures are deeply wired in our brain and have been critical for the survival of our species.[1] Spirituality has long been associated with addiction disorders and the recovery process.[2] More recently, neuroscientists have identified brain structures linked to spiritual and religious experiences.[3] All human beings have neural structures that create and modulate our spirituality.[4] These brain structures create meaning and transcendence. Each one of us is therefore biologically wired for interdependence and transcendent spiritual experiences.

Addiction initially captures our spiritual hunger and feelings, redirecting spirituality unto itself. Over time, this erodes normal spiritual and religious activities or renders them hollow. As if this is not enough, addiction also erodes the ability to maintain healthy connections with others. Relationships are destroyed by dishonesty, deception, and the self-serving characteristics of the disease. Because addiction destroys healthy social connections and one's spiritual qualities, it makes sense that the road to recovery must include repair in these areas. When we look back over more than a century of humankind's battle with addiction, a religious or spiritual quest has been at the center of nearly every victory over addiction. In the same manner, nearly every story that depicts individuals overcoming addiction involves the interconnection with ones' fellows. Very often, this same story describes a transcendent experience. No matter how independent an individual is, learning healthy interdependence is a central part of recovery for most people.

Coaches in team sports have intuitively recognized that when a team works together with mutually reinforcing members, it has a higher probability of success. Research verifies that collective efficiency and team performance have mutually reinforcing effects. That is, teams with high cohesion and collective efficiency increase the probability of success, and this success increases cohesion.[5] This, in turn, increases the psychological health of all teammates.[6] In sharp contrast, the bulk of our educational system is based upon individual achievement and grade performance, the equivalent of social Darwinism.[7] Since our job is to help every patient attain recovery, we must act more like coaches than examiners handing out grades.

In Domain E, work is divided into two parts, interpersonal connectedness and spirituality. They are both a part of Domain E because they are part of the same process, extending outside of oneself, asking for help, and using the connection with others and one's Higher Power to heal. As one progresses in recovery, giving back seems more important. This is often focused on providing help to other individuals who suffer from addiction. The process of "giving back" accelerates addiction repair in the giver and receiver, deepening the commitment to connection and spiritual growth. When working in the group-based elements of treatment, focusing on the collective milieu improves the prognosis for individual patients. The patients under our care are a team, not a collection of individuals.[8] If you are an individual therapist, work in parts of Domain E is more difficult. The therapist should inquire about interactions with support groups, supportive friends, family, and coworkers to help the client develop meaningful relationships.

Attachment and Emotional Regulation

In Domain C, I discussed the coping skills of self-soothing and self-guided emotional regulation. Clinical experience shows that managing difficult emotions may best be accomplished by combining individual skills with interpersonal attachment. First described by Bowlby[9] and defined in addiction disorders by Flores,[10] interpersonal styles of relating or attaching are critical here, specifically for emotional regulation and human development in general.[11] Flores reports that disorders of attachment are central to the development of addiction, and repair of these problems are a necessary step in the recovery process. This repair begins in residential treatment, day treatment, or intensive outpatient treatment and continues with support group meetings and long-term recovery management.

You may already intuitively comprehend the importance of healthy attachment in recovery. Consider patients who have done well in recovery. Such patients often report positive feelings toward therapists, staff, and treatment peers. They report building new friendships in support group meetings and a reconnection with their families. Dr. Flores, in his book *Addiction as an Attachment Disorder*,[10] describes how to build such attachments as part of a robust recovery.

Ainsworth defined four types of childhood attachment: secure, anxious-resistant, anxious-avoidant, and disorganized.[12] These patterns are expressed later in all adult relationships, including romantic relationships. These childhood patterns will therefore express themselves in treatment settings and affect a patient's ability to use interpersonal support and guidance both during and after treatment. During the initial assessment, staff should consider a patient's attachment style, assisting him or her in moving from maladaptive attachment (anxious-resistant, anxious-avoidant, and disorganized) to secure attachment to others and to a peer group. Many patients who are attachment challenged will do better connecting to a group than to individuals within that group. Orderly, structured groups are best; this is where twelve-step support groups shine, with defined meeting times, a predictable sequence, and structured interactions.[10]

Work in Domain E is aimed at overcoming maladaptive attachment styles to the extent that they interfere with our patients' ability to:

- Find and bond with a healthy peer group that entrains non-chemical fun.
- Use guidance from sponsor, therapists, and other members of a support group.
- Trust external advice, especially when it contradicts internal guidance (i.e., AddictBrain thinking).
- Find meaning and feel part of a group.
- Be able to help and experience gratitude from volunteering help to others.
- Decrease shame by sharing personal ethical violations and realizing such violations are a central and universal experience in addiction.
- Provide hope for others and in doing so rediscover hope for oneself.

If a patient suffers from a sufficiently maladaptive interpersonal style, he or she will not be able to accomplish some or all of these goals in early treatment. This is, however, one of the most important tasks in the first two years of recovery. Treatment centers may already do some of this through alumni groups or returning to the center weekly for ongoing support.

All of us in the addiction treatment community are steeped in the dangers of co-addiction (also called codependence). If this is your first introduction to healthy attachment, you may wonder how it is different from codependent relationships. These differences apply to couples, friendships, and other groups, including therapy groups and mutual help groups. Table E1 below outlines the differences.

**Table E1: Differences between Co-Addiction
and Healthy Attachment in Coupleship and in Groups**

Codependent	Healthy Attachment
Imbalance of power among members.	Balance of power among members.
One partner or group member takes on responsibilities of the other(s).	Each member takes responsibility for his or her actions.
Both halves require the other to function.	Members function well independently but achieve a higher level of functioning through group interaction and support.
One member often controls or expresses the feelings of the others.	Although empathy occurs, members of the coupleship or group do not merge feeling states; each experiences his or her own unique reactions to situations.
One individual expresses emotions that are inappropriate or taboo to the other(s).	Members express their own emotions and can express a full range of emotions.

Codependent	Healthy Attachment
Interpersonal growth and exploration are inhibited; it threatens the stability of the group.	Interpersonal growth and exploration is encouraged. The couple or group evolves over time.
Either half of a coupleship or some members (in a group) feel trapped or smothered by the relationship or group.	Members experience an expanding self-awareness.
Group members are threatened by differences.	Differences between members of a group are celebrated and encouraged.
Feelings are for control.	Feelings increase connection without controlling others.
One or both halves feel compelled to fix the other's problems.	Problems are acknowledged and discussed. Advice, encouragement, and support are provided, but the problem remains with the individual.
Boundaries between each other are fused and confused.	Individuals feel a clear sense of self with different feeling states and emotional responses, tastes, skills, and interests.
One-half of a relationship or one member of a group dominates the agenda of others.	Each person in a coupleship or group is drawn together by a common purpose, cause, or passion.
Individuals come together to support a single person or agenda. The power of such a group or couple is less than the sum of the individuals involved.	Members come together and in doing so create a third distinct energy. The resultant synergy creates a power that is greater than the sum of the parts.
Communication is one-sided, often leaving out the ideas, opinions, and dreams of others.	Healthy communication allows all parties to interact and discuss issues that enhances effectiveness and avoids misunderstandings.
The relationship has little tolerance for disruption or distress.	Disruption and distress is handled through mutual problem-solving.
The relationship is stagnant. Any attempt for a member to change is thwarted by the rigid nature of the relationship.	The relationship evolves, mutually enhancing members of the coupleship or group.

Building Spirituality Through Steps Two and Three

At this point in treatment, most patients will have completed Step One (Domain B). In Domain E, we expand the patient's twelve-step work, focusing on Steps Two and Three. By this time, most patients have accepted the illness as being substantive and are open to formulating a path out of illness. This starts with Steps Two and Three. The combination of interpersonal connectedness and connection with a Higher Power of their choosing builds a solid foundation for continued abstinence. Since many addiction therapists have significant experience with the Twelve Steps of Alcoholics Anonymous, I will not expand on them here but instead provide a systematic manner of working with these two steps. You may wish to refresh your knowledge by reading Steps Two and Three in the "Twelve and Twelve."[13] In addition, review the steps as described in the AA Big Book[14] and the NA Basic Text.[15] Many guides to step work are available for consultation as well.[16]

Table E2: Principles Behind Steps Two and Three

Step		Character Problem	Principle	Action
2	Came to believe that a Power greater than ourselves could restore us to sanity.	Self will and disbelief	Hope	Realization
3	Made a decision to turn our will and our lives over to the care of God, as we understood Him.	Self-will and fear	Faith	Ask for and accept help

Many patients will rediscover or explore the religious or spiritual teachings of their youth during this period of treatment. Therapists and staff should avoid using any pressure in this regard. Spiritual and religious beliefs are very personal and, at the same time, powerful for many. If staff members hold strong beliefs, they have the potential to temporarily nudge patients into one belief system or another. The patient, in an effort to "do the correct thing" may respond with false compliance that hinders a more genuine examination of his or her own personal spiritual path.

Domain E focuses primarily on the interpersonal connectedness aspects of spirituality and on the emotional regulation this involves. It has three Skills Groups:

E1) Practicing Group Healing

E2) Group-Based Problem-Solving

E3) Building Trust

Domain E has four worksheets:

E1) The **How Others Help Our Recovery** Worksheet. This worksheet is completed and discussed in Assignment Group (task E1). It builds healthy interdependence in the group and increased gratitude for all.

E2) The **Step Two** Worksheet. This worksheet helps patients explore and commit to Step Two of Alcoholics Anonymous.

E3) The **Step Three** Worksheet. This worksheet clarifies a patient's relationship and moves them ahead in Step Three.

E4) The **Helping Others** Worksheet. This worksheet examines the nature of giving. It requires a willingness on the part of the patient to engage in through self-examination and may not be right for everyone. Patients who are especially codependent or self-castigating can find quite a bit of relief if they have the capacity for self-forgiveness.

There are four Assignment Group tasks in Domain E:

E1) Sharing the worksheet: **How Others Help Our Recovery**. This assignment helps the protagonist experience connection and gratitude. It teaches him or her to validate others and deepens connections to peers in recovery.

E2) Discussing the worksheet for **Step Two**. Working through Step Two in Assignment Group helps the protagonist explore his or her reactions to work on Step Two.

E3) Discussing the worksheet for **Step Three**. When shared in Assignment Group, this difficult step is examined and clarified. When a patient takes on this task in Assignment Group, he or she is taking Step Three to the best of his or her ability. This Assignment Group task is practice for later work with an AA sponsor. As with all tasks related to the Twelve Steps, patients learn that this task prepares them for working this step with their sponsor at some future date.

E4) Sharing the **Helping Others** worksheet. This painful revealing assignment digs into the nature of giving and in doing so the importance of caring for others to further one's own recovery.

Domain E: Skills Groups

Skills Group E1: Practicing Group Healing

A substantial part of the evolution from addiction to recovery is built on group effort. I often tell patients, "We don't know why this is, but group therapy and structured group meetings are the most effective way to recover from addiction." This does not mean that recovery never occurs when an individual works alone or with just one other human being. This happens but is not the norm. Despite this fact, treatment organizations commonly do not help clients understand this basic goal of group therapy nor do they instruct them how to use group work to heal. Domain E does just that.

In Skills Group E1, patients are taught some of the many skills for group work and, most importantly, they practice those skills with real time encouragement and feedback. The skills taught in E1 (which may extend over many sessions if need be) are many. Members of this (these) Skills Groups teach patients how to:

- Express appreciation to others
- Tell others when they are feeling misunderstood
- Achieve understanding though group interaction
- Express fear and a lack of safety when this pops up in group
- Express negative emotions without attacking or feeling judged
- Bring up a topic that is difficult or painful

- Support the feelings of others without hijacking the group process onto themselves
- Confront another patient on maladaptive thoughts or behaviors effectively
- Accept healthy confrontation without feeling belittled or shamed

This is a grand list, but every element will not be achieved overnight, especially when we consider how broken many of our patients are when they arrive. We encourage staff who work with this Skills Group to pick one or two of the current issues in the group and start the practice there. For example, if on the previous day a patient harshly confronted another patient and that second patient angrily shut down or left the group therapy, the following day is a good time to work on healthy confrontation. If the group makes progress on that skill, the leader may suggest a second area to build on the first.

Therapists tend to overlap this Skills Group with Process Group. I think this is ill advised, especially when patients arrive in a group without previous experience. In early treatment, shifting from skill-building to unstructured Process Groups is difficult. True unstructured process work is scary and difficult; this is one important reason why Process Groups inadvertently regress into superficial and dispassionate discussion.

Domain E teaches these skills within a formal framework. The most important technique of this Skills Group is to move slowly carefully asking the protagonist(s) what he or she feels and encouraging group feedback gently and repeatedly. Let us pick one example: *Accepting healthy confrontation without feeling belittled or shamed.* The leader may recall an event from a previous group where Jane was confronted when she blamed her spouse, "He makes me drink." Thinking back, the leader remembers the confrontation as direct and a bit harsh, but accurate. The leader gently asks Jane if they can use this event as a way of helping all of them to accept feedback, even painful feedback from others. Rather than replay that event (and hoping for a different outcome), the leader generalizes the problem: "All of us have difficulties with tough feedback, don't we?"

Jane agrees to become the protagonist. The leader immediately asks her to enroll a double. Jane will instruct the double what she should say and how she feels. The leader instructs the protagonist, Jane, to pick someone in the group to enroll as the individual who confronted her previously. It is important to avoid selecting the confronter to play him- or herself. These individuals may be placed at the center of the group facing each other (or preferably at a less provocative sixty-degree angle). Jane describes and asks her double to experience her emotions before the confrontation. She then instructs the confronter actor to say what she thought she heard. Moving back and forth from confronter to her double, she plays out the scene. The leader stops the action at critical moments, requesting group feedback. Feedback should not be "No, it was not like that, it happened like this . . ." The goal is not to correct the past; it is to understand what is occurring in the room at present.

If Jane feels safe and provides permission, the leader brings in the person or persons who provided the past confrontation. The confronter (we will call him Jim) becomes the next protagonist. Jim plays out the past event as he remembers it. The leader starts and stops the action requesting refinements in the confrontation scene that will help both individuals work together, learning how to listen without fighting back or falling into a pit of self-flagellation and shame.

If the leader has sufficient training in experiential therapy, he or she may find it helpful to bring in Jane and Jim's historical figures that are the foundation of the current situation. For example, Jim may have had a father who said, "A man says the truth and lets the chips fall where they may." Jane may have had parents who shamed mercilessly for numerous insignificant imperfections.

The goal of this scene is to help both protagonists (and by extension all group members) learn how to be direct in confrontation and, at the same time, respect and sidestep shaming behaviors. When the leader stops and starts action, the entire group participates in healing itself. Once the initial scene has been properly worked through, a member may suggest a possible solution during an interruption in the action. The leader asks Jane and Jim, "Can we try the interaction that was just suggested?" This helps all members see that group is an experiment in living a way of practicing alternative interpersonal styles.

Skills Group E2: Group-Based Problem-Solving

The purpose of this group is learning how to problem solve in a group. Members learn how to set aside individual bias, listen to others, accept changes and improvements to preconceived notions and, ultimately, to recognize that a collective solution is often superior to individual problem-solving. Along the way, clients will uncover solutions to common recovery dilemmas.

The goal of this Skills Group is to have everyone learn the benefits of group-based problem-solving. In this Skills Group, the leader picks out between three and five individuals who role-play a small group within the group. They move their chairs inside, producing a circle within a circle. The leader also reasserts the importance of learning how to work cooperatively with others as a means of ensuring solid and sustainable recovery.

The interior members are tasked with solving several situations that could potentially lead to relapse. The leader begins with a predefined, high-risk situation. If this situation falls flat or is quickly processed, the leader may ask the exterior members to suggest a difficult future situation for the interior group to process.

Note that the leader's job is to refocus the group repeatedly on healthy group therapy problem-solving. The actual solution of the given situation is of lesser importance. Toward these ends, the leader stops and starts the protagonists' interactions in the inner circle. If one protagonist ignores or discounts another protagonist's input, the leader stops the problem-solving process asking members of the outside circle to comment on what just happened. At this point, members of the outer circle offer constructive feedback to the problem-solving process occurring in the inner circle. Less often, members of the inner circle may themselves comment and correct. When an issue has solved, the protagonists who occupied the inner circle resumes their problem solving.

Several common trends repeatedly appear in this Skills Group format. A member often attempts to control the discussion or offer advice using an authoritative tone. The Skills Group leader carefully watches other group members when this occurs, looking to see if the self-appointed expert's approach (often dogmatic or controlling) shuts down additional discussion. If so, the leader stops the process and asks members of the outer circle to comment on what happened. Occasionally, one member may take a fatalistic or pessimistic stance, torpedoing constructive ideas. This, too, is commented upon by the outer circle. Protagonists are encouraged to avoid overly simplistic and singular conclusions. If a group of protagonists comes up with a direct solution in a few minutes, the leader then asks, "What are some other possible solutions to this situation?" If the inner circle has used group-based problem-solving well, the leader can increase the complexity of the recovery dilemma, adding additional stressors to the situation. These additional elements increase the stress associated with problem-solving in the inner circle and thus increase discussion about effective group-based problem-solving.

When this Skills Group is functioning at its best, members of the outer circle raise a hand or carefully interject a question for the protagonists in the inner circle to consider. It is extremely important to stop members of the outer circle from interjecting advice. Their job is to comment on the process of the group solution, not to offer solutions themselves. If members of the outer circle fall into solving the (sham) problem posed to the inner circle, this Skills Group breaks down rapidly and its goal is lost. Therefore, the leader should immediately intervene with a brief reeducation when this inevitably happens.

Once a pre-constructed recovery dilemma has been solved, the leader reselects members for the inner group. The leader may ask for a specific recovery dilemma to be the subject of problem-solving in the next scene.

Here is one possible pre-constructed recovery dilemma.

> *John is out of town on a business trip. He is ninety days into recovery and to date has had*
> *very few problems in maintaining his abstinence from alcohol. Part of his work is taking*
> *potential customers out to dinner. He has had a regular relationship with many of these*
> *customers and feels reasonably comfortable with them. For his first trip out of town, he*
> *goes to dinner with two customers he knows well. On this trip, however, his two customers*
> *brought along three other individuals John does not know. His two longtime customers like*
> *John and are trying to be helpful by introducing John to additional business.*

> *As usual, John takes his customers to a relatively nice restaurant that serves alcohol.*
> *Although he feels his older two customers are friends, he is too embarrassed to let them*
> *know about his recovery status and he fears their disapproval. He does not want to lose*
> *their business. John has not met the three potential customers who are coming along.*
> *At dinner, John quickly discovers that at least two of the new customers are heavy drinkers*
> *and unfortunately are the type of drinkers who want everyone to imbibe with them. They*
> *begin to pester John about having a drink with them, commenting with mild derision about*
> *his sparkling water with lime. In doing so, they insinuate that he is "a lightweight" with a*
> *tone that questions his masculinity.*

> *What should John do?*

Skills Group E3: Building Trust

In this Skills Group, the leader explores trust with others. Requirements of this exercise are two rooms (or if weather permits, one room and an outside area) and two blindfolds. Before the group starts, the leader randomly places chairs or other obstacles about in room 1 (or outside). It is best to have these obstacles tightly placed; creating a tortuous path that is difficult to traverse. This is the Recovery Maze.

Patients and the leader first meet in room 2 where chairs are placed in a conventional circle. The leader explains the purpose of the group: groups work best if members trust each other. One patient is identified as the first protagonist. The protagonist identifies another member as a support figure; this individual can enroll as a sponsor, mentor, or other metaphor that works for the protagonist. It is best to use generic terms and avoid the baggage that would arise if historical figures were used (historical figures also take the protagonist out of the group and defeat the purpose of this exercise). The leader should consider bypassing members for the protagonist role who are victims of past ritualized trauma, but such individuals often feel empowered by acting as a support figure in this exercise. The support figure comes to the protagonist and gently blindfolds the protagonist. They then gently place hands on the protagonist's shoulder helping him or her stand. The protagonist is guided to the maze and informed when he or she enters. To do this, the support figure stands directly behind or aside the protagonist, with a hand gently on each shoulder. The protagonist is guided by gentle pressure on either shoulder and with frequent quiet words of encouragement.

Other group members quietly walk into the room and place themselves about the room. They collectively enroll as the "voice of addiction" or "AddictBrain." At first, these voices are quiet or murmur imperceptibly. The leader guides comment volume and intensity. The protagonist begins a very slow walk through the room with his support figure guiding by using firm but gentle pressure on his or her shoulders or by using brief verbal guidance, such as, "walk two steps forward then turn left." When the enrolled voices of addiction do speak, they do so individually at first, contradicting the protagonist's guidance through the maze ("No that is wrong, it will be much more fun if you go to your left!"). As the experience builds, the leader may ask the addiction voices to discount the support voice (e.g., "Whoa, this guy is sending you the wrong way!" or "No, walk in the other direction!"). If the protagonist can tolerate it, the leader has the AddictBrain voices begin to speak all together, issuing contradictory commands.

When the protagonist has traversed the room (or had enough), the voices of addiction disenroll as a group. The support figure walks the protagonist out of the maze and back to the group room, where he or she disenrolls. It is best to keep the protagonist blindfolded until he or she returns to room 2. Everyone sits and the group processes the experience. The leader asks the protagonist to decompress first. The group discusses how the exercise is or is not like being addicted. If time permits, additional group participants take on the protagonist role, and the process repeats.

Domain E: Assignment Groups Tasks

Assignment Group Task E1: How Others Help

In this Assignment Group, patients learn how to connect with each other through mutual help and sharing. The primary methodology used in this group is through the sharing of gratitude, which expands on existing gratitude in the giver and receiver.[17] The process of expanding group gratitude is hidden in the sharing of Worksheet E1. Here, the protagonist reads a list of ways others have helped him or her in his or her recovery. This Assignment Group teaches the reader about the benefits that come from expressing gratitude. This exercise increased caring between all members and the gratitude among its members. It also deepens interdependence among group members. This in turn increases hope and serves as a model each patient can use in his or her family and support network.

Assignment Group Task E2: Step Two

In this group task, the protagonist reviews his or her Step Two Worksheet. The leader asks the client to read the contents of the worksheet, stopping frequently for clarifications and discussion. It is important to avoid having the protagonist just read through his or her responses to worksheet questions. It is also important to have group members keep an open mind about the varieties of religious and spiritual beliefs that may be present in the room. Proselytizing should be avoided at all costs.

Assignment Group Task E3: Step Three

This group task is like E2 above. As with the task related to Step Two, participants are cautioned against preaching cultural, religious, or spiritual beliefs to others. Everyone, including the protagonist, is encouraged to keep an open mind during this exercise. Group participants are encouraged to avoid advice giving; sharing of experiences proves to be more helpful during this task.

Assignment Group Task E4: Helping Others

This Assignment Group task should only be performed in a setting where group members have sufficient maturity and low judgmentalism. The protagonist who reads from Worksheet E4 should also be able to describe his or her shortcomings rather than using this task as a way of self-aggrandizement. The group leader needs to be able to take the pulse of the group, constantly shifting back and forth between decreasing hostility and increasing the protagonist's honest appraisal of his or her past giving behaviors.

When properly executed this Assignment Group task can encourage deep sharing of regrets and help shift all members from self-serving to mutual assistance.

Domain E: Connectedness and Spirituality Worksheets

Overview of Worksheets

Worksheets in Domain E accomplish four goals: seeking help from a Higher Power, learning to use groups for personal growth, developing healthy interdependency, and rearranging values toward service and helping others.

There are four worksheets in Domain E:

E1) The **How Others Help** Worksheet. Patients who complete this worksheet are reviewing how other patients in treatment have promoted their health and recovery. The individual who completes this worksheet learns to recognize and acknowledge how others provide recovery assistance. Patients catalog specifically how they could not do it alone, fostering healthy interdependence. When this worksheet is reviewed in Assignment Group, the acknowledgment deepens group cohesiveness. The recipient, in turn, learns to accept gratitude and reflect on how acknowledgment increases interpersonal connection.

E2) The **Step Two** Worksheet. This worksheet walks the patient through Step Two of Alcoholics Anonymous (and related programs).

E3) The **Step Three** Worksheet. This worksheet assists the patient in completing Step Three of Alcoholics Anonymous (and related programs).

E4) The **Helping Others** Worksheet. This brief worksheet establishes a patient's short- and long-term goals regarding service work. It clarifies how service work helps the giver as much as the receiver.

Worksheet E1: How Others Help Our Recovery

Staying in recovery is something that no one could do alone. Many people have tried to go their own way, making ultimatums to themselves, proclamations to others, and coming up with grand schemes to stop the relentless progression of the disease. Over the long run, this seems to fall away. A twelve-step program saying is "Recovery is a WE program not a ME program."

This worksheet helps you catalog and remember the little things (and maybe not so little things) that others have done for you that you cannot do for yourself. You may need to complete this worksheet over a series of weeks. Take your time, returning to it often when someone in your community says or does something for you that increases your insight, reduces your shame, or increases your recovery resolve. Write down a complete description of what occurred in column ①. In column ②, note who helped you. The most important column in this worksheet is column ③. Carefully analyze what happened. Determine exactly why this was something you could not do for yourself. Think carefully here. It may be that you are too proud, did not understand something, or needed external validation for something you yourself could not create. Enter this information into column ③. If you get stumped, look at the list at the end of this worksheet for ways people help each other in recovery.

① What did they do?	② Who helped?	③ How was this something you yourself could not do by yourself?

① What did they do?	② Who helped?	③ How was this something you yourself could not do by yourself?

Bid for time in Assignment Group to review this worksheet, to express your gratitude to others, and to receive feedback.

Here is a list of ways people help each other along the path from addiction to recovery. Use this list to jog your memory about how others have helped you in your recovery. Do not simply copy items from this list onto the worksheet—this would keep this exercise from being meaningful. Use your own words.

Someone helped me with recovery when he or she:

- Became a friend who would do things with me and stay sober with me.
- Reached out his or her hand when I needed it the most.
- Helped me understand a principle or concept that I did not understand.
- Helped me feel less alone.
- Described an event from his or her life that made me feel less shame about what I had done.
- Gave me hope that I could recover.
- Helped me see that group was safe and my peers wanted to help.
- Taught me how to have fun without using.
- Helped me laugh at myself.
- Seemed really concerned about what I was feeling or experiencing.
- Helped me understand or work the steps of AA, NA, CA, or other fellowships.
- Counseled me to do the right thing even though it was difficult.
- Helped me "tell on myself."
- Shared his or her pain and helped me endure my own.
- Helped me feel difficult emotions.
- Showed me how to express a feeling I was taught not to feel or express.
- Helped me feel less alone.
- Showed me how I was fooling myself or lying to myself.
- Showed me how to be compassionate to others.
- Taught me a healthy coping skill.
- Helped me learn a sport or exercise regime.
- Urged me on in group when I had to talk about something difficult.
- Urged me on when trying something new and healthy.
- Gave me a second chance.
- Taught me how to thank others.

Worksheet E2: Step Two

This worksheet walks you through Step Two of the twelve-step program.

Step Two: *Came to believe that a power greater than ourselves could restore us to sanity.*

Before you begin this worksheet read Step Two in *Twelve Steps and Twelve Traditions*. This step is easy for some people and difficult for others. Don't worry if you have never thought about the spiritual aspects of life before. This step is one of exploration and reflection. If you have had a strong spiritual or religious upbringing, this step may be a recommitment to your past values.

The basic elements of Step Two are:
- Accepting that your addiction controlled you in the past and led you to misinterpretations of reality and insane thoughts and behaviors.
- Concluding that you cannot fix the problem on your own.
- Searching for a Higher Power that will help restore sanity to your life.

Some concepts in Step Two are difficult for many people. The first is the notion that your addiction caused you to be insane. *Insane* is a strong word. It may be helpful to remember Step One where you realized that you were powerless over your addiction and your life had become unmanageable. Being powerless and having an unmanageable life is really a form of insanity. Step Two returns to these realizations, asking you to consider how crazy you had become and how AddictBrain took control over parts or all your life.

Question 1: List some of the crazy things you have done in the service of your addiction. _____

_____

_____

Can you comfortably say that you had become insane? ☐ Yes   ☐ No

If you do not feel comfortable stating that your addiction made you out of control and insane, at this moment, that is okay. Stop working on this worksheet and let your therapist know.

Question 2: Consider the times where you have tried to change your use pattern, tried to stop using, or attempted to diminish the negative consequences of your addiction and related beliefs and actions. Were you truly successful on your own for any sustained period? If **yes**, describe how you **were successful** in decreasing use, stopping use, or improving the consequences of your addiction.

_____

_____

_____

If you were **not successful** describe some of those attempts here. _____

_____

_____

_____

Can you comfortably state that you cannot have long-term success without a power outside of yourself?
☐ Yes   ☐ No

If you do not feel comfortable stating that you need a power outside of yourself at this time, then that is okay. Stop working on this worksheet, and let your therapist know. Do not complete this form just to get it done. It is most important that this decision is meaningful.

Question 3: List several powers outside of you that have helped you in the past or you believe might be the most helpful in the future in overcoming your addiction. Consider the love of your family, your spiritual or religious faith, God or any other religious power, the strength of your support system, and any other external power from which you can derive benefit. Remember that Step Two says, "Came to believe that . . ." and does not say, "Came to believe **in** . . ." This means that the extent of your faith in any of the powers at this moment of time need only be that they will restore sanity. Deeper faith may come in time.

List each power in column ①. Then, go back and rank by how acceptable they are to you (1 is highly acceptable and 5 not acceptable) in column ②. Finally, rank how effective each of these powers will be in helping you recover. Rate them from 1 to the total number of entries, 1 being the most effective.

① Powers Outside of Myself That Will Help Me with Sobriety	② Acceptable/ Not Acceptable	③ Rank (1 is Highest)

Many of us have mixed feelings about the religion of our family. Think about how you feel about your childhood and your family's religious training. It may help to write about it in Question 4 below.

Question 4: List the positive and negative aspects of your family's religion as you see it today.

Positive: _____

_____

_____

_____

Negative: _____

_____

_____

_____

Set this worksheet aside. You will present it in Assignment Group. After that presentation, you will return to answer the question below.

Question 5: Have you come to believe that a Higher Power could restore you to sanity?

☐ Yes   ☐ No   ☐ I need to think about this for a while before taking this step.

For now, my Higher Power will be: _____

Worksheet E3: Step Three

This worksheet walks you through Step Three of the twelve-step program.

Step Three: Made a decision to turn our will and our lives over to the care of God as we understood Him.

Before you begin this worksheet, read Step Three in the *Twelve Steps and Twelve Traditions*. This step requires action like most of the steps of the twelve-step program. Many people have trouble with the absolute quality of the action implied in this step. How can you completely turn your will over to a Higher Power? Will you become a zombie or drone? Will you lose the ability to make decisions? Will you lose yourself in this venture? In time, you will find that none of these come to pass.

The Twelve Steps and Twelve Traditions talks about opening the door to Step Three using the key of willingness. It is often best to make the decision to try Step Three and then to turn over pieces of your life a bit at a time. You may be amazed at the results.

The elements of Step Three are:
- Acknowledging that you have not done the best possible job managing your life.
- Listing specific parts of your life that need help.
- Search for the willingness to turn part or all your life over to the Higher Power you named in Worksheet E2.

Question 1: List a few of the parts of your life where you need help, parts where your willpower and decisions have caused you significant problems. _____

_____

_____

_____

Question 2: Do you have problems trusting others or have you been betrayed or hurt by powers outside of yourself? If so, list what happened in the past here. _____

_____

_____

_____

Question 3: List some things in your life on which you have become dependent. Consider modern conveniences (electricity, automobiles, and traffic control systems, heating, computers, and the internet).

_____

_____

_____

Are you "dependent" on these things and do you put your trust in them in that they will help you navigate your everyday life? ☐ Yes   ☐ No

Question 4a: Describe how you **have** turned your will and your life over to AddictBrain in the past:

_____

_____

Question 4b: Describe how you **have not** turned your will and your life over to AddictBrain in the past:

_____

_____

Question 5: Review your answers to Questions 1 through 4 above. When you consider problems generated by your addiction and any past difficulties with control or trust, can you accept outside help with your addiction?   ☐ Yes   ☐ No

If yes, describe how this is true for you: _____

_____

_____

_____

If no, describe why this is not true for you: _____

_____

_____

_____

Question 6a: Assume that you turn control your addiction and your life over to the Higher Power of your understanding. In what ways might this result in a life with more independence than you have had when addicted? _____

_____

_____

_____

Question 6b: Assume that you **do not** turn control your addiction over to your Higher Power. In what ways will you have more independence than if you did? _____

_____

_____

_____

Question 6c: Can you see how turning your addiction over to you Higher Power may result in having a life that is more in control than out of control?   ☐ Yes   ☐ No

If you do not feel comfortable stating that turning your addiction over to a power outside of yourself will help, that is OK. Stop working on this worksheet and let your therapist know. Do not complete this form just to get it done. It is more important that this decision is meaningful.

Question 7: Reviewing your answers above and after careful reflection, decide which of the following applies to you. Choose the one answer that best describes your thoughts and beliefs right now.

☐ Right now, I cannot turn anything over to a power greater than myself or there is no power greater than myself.

☐ I have limited trust in anything outside of myself but will work on building trust.

☐ I can turn over my treatment to professionals but cannot turn my recovery or anything else over to any outside powers.

☐ I can turn over my willpower but only regarding my addiction. I will turn this over to this Higher Power: _____

☐ I can turn most things in my life over to a Higher Power, that power being: _____

☐ Right now, I cannot turn over my will power in these areas: _____

_____

_____

☐ I am completely ready to turn my will and my life over to the care of my Higher Power. I call this power _____.

Question 8: Review your answer to Question 7 above. What might help you move from your checked answer to the next item down the list?

_____

_____

_____

Worksheet E4: Helping Others

In this worksheet you take stock of how you have helped others. You will examine your motives and actions, looking for selfless service to others. During addiction therapy you spend a lot of time looking at what you have done wrong. This worksheet, in contrast, validates helpful actions, kindness, and assistance you have selflessly provided to others—to acknowledge your goodness and compassion.

Many of you will be surprised at how available you have been to your friends, family, benevolent organizations, or even strangers. Recording these efforts will boost your self-esteem during times of rigorous and often painful self-reflection. Be aware, however, that this worksheet may also shine the light on acts of philanthropy that may not have been as selfless as you first thought.

Recovery teaches individuals that when they give of themselves, they gain inner strength and peace. By the same token, when you give with your own agenda, if it is more for yourself than for others, and it erodes inner peace and hardens the heart.

Fill out column ① below first by listing times you have helped others. Make a comprehensive list without thinking about the reasons for your actions. Then, go back through the list and analyze your giving into one of the categories below. Enter this in column ②.

Here are the types of giving:

> **C – Codependent** giving. This means giving to others when doing so zaps your own energy, makes your life worse, or the giving causes you to lose sight of self-care.

> **S – Selfish** giving. Giving to others in such a manner that you feed your ego or wind up giving because you will get more in return. Boastful giving falls into this category.

> **R – Required** giving. This type of giving occurs because your role in life demands that you do so. If your giving is required by your role (a parent providing a home and safety to a child) then place an R in this item *unless you believe that your giving was done with a loving and an open spirit most of the time.* If a role-dependent giving has these qualities it should be coded as SL(see below).

> **SL – Selfless** giving. Selfless giving is done out of the kindness of your heart, expecting nothing in return. Most anonymous giving falls in this category.

For many in recovery, this exercise is at least a bit painful. Be honest and thorough and avoid judging yourself. Remember this exercise can open the door to change and provide you the means to do so. Exposing past giving as **C**, **S**, or **R** will clarify your actions later and set you free from confusing acts of kindness.

Now go through the list a third time, filling out column ③. You may not need to enter anything in column ③ if the giving type was selfless (SL). Reconsider your relationship with giving behaviors. Do you drain your energy with C (codependent) giving? Do you appear to be extraordinarily kind when most of your giving is C (selfish)? The hollow results can be improved by increasing SL (selfless) giving. Discuss this in group.

Question 1: The nature of giving

① What did you do to help others?	② Giving type	③ How could the giving have been done differently?

① What did you do to help others?	② Giving type	③ How could the giving have been done differently?

Question 2: If you labeled any giving as C above, what were the qualities of this giving that wound up being problematic or counterproductive to you? _____

_____

_____

_____

Question 3: List one or more times where you have helped others while in treatment. _____

_____

_____

_____

_____

Question 4: Describe your plans for one future episode of selfless giving. _____

_____

_____

_____

_____

Domain E: Progress Assessment Form

RecoveryMind Training – Connectedness and Spirituality

Domain E Recovery Skill	Date: Patient B	I	C	Staff B	I	C	Date: Patient B	I	C	Staff B	I	C	Date: Patient B	I	C	Staff B	I	C
Is able to recognize how others help with goal attainment and personal growth.																		
Is able to recognize help from others and express gratitude at some a later date.																		
Is able to recognize how others are giving to him or her and can express gratitude at the time help has been provided.																		
Has completed Worksheet E2 (Step Two) and received feedback in Assignment Group.																		
Has internalized Step Two.																		
Has completed Worksheet E3 (Step Three) and received feedback in Assignment Group.																		
Has internalized Step Three and has implemented it in his or her daily life.																		
Understands the different types of giving (Codependent, Selfish, Required, and Selfless).																		
Can recognize and differentiate his or her giving to others in the past and correctly properly categorize the same.																		
Has plans for future selfless giving to others.																		
Has practiced selfless giving to others in his or her treatment community and/or family unit.																		

This evaluation is completed by both the patient or client (self-assessment) and his or her therapist or staff members on this one form. After starting work on a skill, place the approximate start date in the column provided. The patient or client fills out the form first. A therapist or staff member performs the same evaluation, placing a check mark in each row that indicates progress in assigned Recovery Skills. This process may need to be repeated for a several times as work progresses in each domain.

A check mark in the **B** column signifies that work has begun. The **I** column should be checked if the patient is in an intermediate or midway through his or her work on this item, and the **C** column should be checked if the patient has made sufficient progress in the skill to move forward to his or her next task. Review and discussion of this form helps patients and therapists set clear treatment expectations and recovery goals.

Domain E: Connectedness and Spirituality Notes

1. R. Adolphs. "The Neurobiology of Social Cognition." *Curr Opin Neurobiol* 11, no. 2 (2001): 231–39.

2. M. Galanter. "Spirituality and Addiction: A Research and Clinical Perspective." *The American Journal on Addictions* 15, no. 4 (2006): 286–92.

3. A. B. Newberg, and E. G. d'Aquili. "The Neuropsychology of Religious and Spiritual Experience." *Journal of Consciousness Studies* 7, no. 11-12 (2000): 251–66.

4. E. Mohandas. "Neurobiology of Spirituality." *Mens sana monographs* 6, no. 1 (2008): 63.

5. J. P. Heuzé, N. Raimbault, and P. Fontayne. "Relationships between Cohesion, Collective Efficacy and Performance in Professional Basketball Teams: An Examination of Mediating Effects." *J Sports Sci* 24, no. 1 (2006): 59–68.

6. D. W. Johnson, R. T. Johnson, and M. L. Krotee. "The Relation between Social Interdependence and Psychological Health on the 1980 US Olympic Ice Hockey Team." *The Journal of Psychology* 120, no. 3 (1986): 279–91.

7. D. W. Johnson, R. T. Johnson, and E. Holubec. *Cooperation in the Classroom.* 8 ed. Edina, MN: Interaction Book Company, 2008.

8. G. D. Leon. "Therapeutic Communities for Addictions: A Theoretical Framework." *Subst Use Misuse* 30, no. 12 (1995): 1603–45.

9. M. S. Ainsworth, and J. Bowlby. "An Ethological Approach to Personality Development." *American Psychologist* 46, no. 4 (1991): 333–41.

10. P. J. Flores. *Addiction as an Attachment Disorder.* Oxford: Jason Aronson, Inc., 2004.

11. H. F. Harlow, and S. J. Suomi. "Social Recovery by Isolation-Reared Monkeys." *Proceedings of the National Academy of Sciences* 68, no. 7 (1971): 1534–38.

12. M. D. Ainsworth, M. Blehar, E. Waters, and S. Wall. *Patterns of Attachment: A Psychological Study of the Strange Situation.* Hillsdale, NJ: Lawrence Erlbaum, 1978.

13. Alcoholics Anonymous World Services. *Twelve Steps and Twelve Traditions.* New York: AA World Services, 2002.

14. A. A. World Services. *Alcoholics Anonymous.* 4th ed. New York: A.A. World Services, 2013.

15. Narcotics Anonymous. *Narcotics Anonymous Basic Text.* Sixth Edition ed.: Narcotics Anonymous World Services, Inc., 2008.

16. P. Carnes. *A Gentle Path through the Twelve Steps: The Classic Guide for All People in the Process of Recovery.* Third ed.: Hazelden, 2012.

17. K. M. Sheldon, and S. Lyubomirsky. "How to Increase and Sustain Positive Emotion: The Effects of Expressing Gratitude and Visualizing Best Possible Selves." *The Journal of Positive Psychology* 1, no. 2 (2006): 73–82.

Domain F: Relapse Prevention
Skills Groups, Assignments, Worksheets, and the Progress Assessment Form

Chapter Overview

Domain F teaches and provides a framework for practicing relapse prevention techniques. Note all domains provide relapse prevention strategies. What Domain F provides are specific skills whose sole purpose is relapse prevention. Individuals can begin this work at any time during treatment, but many of the strategies detailed here are most effective when the client has a clear grasp of what he or she is up against. The worksheets can be completed and reviewed in individual therapy as well as organized treatment; however, the Skills Groups can only be effectively taught in a group therapy setting, regardless of where the group occurs—residential settings, outpatient therapy, or adjunctive therapy in a recovery residence are all fine. Keep in mind that those patients who are triggered or otherwise at a high risk of relapse may require containment due to the triggering effect of some of these exercises.

Definitions

Terms vary widely throughout addiction medicine; this is especially so when discussing relapse and its prevention. RecoveryMind Training has specific definitions and uses conventions when working on relapse prevention. I do not claim they are more exacting than other nomenclature schemes. However, RecoveryMind Training emphatically believes that consistency of language is extremely important in what we do as clinicians—it creates clarity for clients who are in a befuddled condition. Therefore, the therapist (or all staff in organized treatment) should become familiar with these definitions and use them in a consistent fashion. RMT is exacting about definitions and terms. This helps patients or clients develop a deep cohesive understanding of addiction. Some of the important terms relating to relapse prevention appear below.

> **Trigger:** Triggers are brain events that instigate thoughts or emotions related to substance procurement, use, or consequences. Triggers often introduce cravings but do not necessarily do so. Another term for "trigger" is "cue." The goal of trigger management is to catalog the myriad brain events that elicit them, coming up with simple behavioral techniques to prevent them from escalating into cravings. Triggers are generated by four sources: environmental triggers, visceral events (body sensations, taste, or smell), emotional events (a feeling that the person with an alcohol use disorder "used to drink over"), and memory tapes (scenes that play in the mind, especially those with strong visual "tapes").

Triggers cannot be avoided. The process of delineating triggers and developing appropriate responses to them improves a client's competence in managing them when they inevitably occur in the future.

Craving: Craving is defined as an intense, urgent, or abnormal desire or longing. According to RecoveryMind Training, cravings can be overt or covert. Overt cravings are recognized as such by their victim. Covert cravings are unconscious. When cravings are beneath awareness, they induce behaviors that lead to alcohol or other drug procurement or set the patient directly on the path to relapse in the behavioral addiction without conscious recognition of the craving—at least initially. Overt cravings have qualities of urgency, intensity, duration, recurrence, and persistence. The most destructive cravings also have qualities of inevitability (they feel as if they will continue mercilessly and can only be solved by relapse). One object of cravings management is make covert cravings overt so they can be managed and relapse prevented.

Relapse: It may seem obvious what a relapse is, but clarity is important when considering this term. Pulling directly from the *Merriam-Webster* Dictionary, relapse is defined as "a recurrence of symptoms of a disease after a period of improvement." One subtlety arises with the phrase *after a period of improvement*. Using this definition, if a patient walks out of a brief treatment and directly enters a bar to get drunk, he or she has not relapsed. Such an individual has not had a period of improvement; recovery had not yet taken hold. Such an incident is best described as a need for more treatment (or a treatment failure) rather than a relapse.

RecoveryMind Training teaches that many symptoms of addiction continue long into recovery. For example, an individual may have nagging and persistent cravings for years. Cravings are clear biological symptoms of addiction. However, RecoveryMind Training does not consider these symptoms as indicative of relapse. This may seem obvious; however, more subtle differentiations exist. Consider an individual with a methamphetamine use disorder who has attained six months of recovery. One day, he gets in his car and drives to his dealer's house with the intention of buying meth. The dealer is not home. Despite deliberate drug-seeking behavior (a significant symptom of addiction[1]), this, too, would not be considered a relapse using RMT nomenclature. Such an individual is indeed at risk for future relapse. His recovery is quite unstable. However, RecoveryMind Training differentiates this as a high-risk situation, not a relapse.

Let's examine the association of these terms more closely. Triggers have the potential for inducing cravings. Cravings, in turn, induce behaviors that place the individual in a high-risk situation, which can result in relapse. Patients may state, "I did not have anything triggering me, I just had a craving." Such statements reflect careless analysis by the client. He or she may see triggers as external things in the environment, minimizing the impact of his or her emotions, memories, or visceral events. In such a case, the relapse prevention therapist should instruct the client to scan through the event, looking for potential trigger suspects. The therapist also has learned that this patient needs additional relapse prevention work. The patient may have larger difficulties with self-examination as well.

In Domain F, a patient's relapse vulnerability can be worked through in its natural sequence. The therapist or staff will start by exploring triggers, move on to learning cravings management, and complete relapse prevention work with a process-oriented relapse prevention model pioneered by Dr. Alan Marlatt.

Identifying and Managing Triggers

Triggers come from any of the human senses (sound, touch, sight, smell, and taste) as well as internal body sensations, emotions, thoughts, and memories. Each recovering individual has his or her own set of triggers and an individual reactivity to these triggers. How powerful they are in stimulating drug seeking and drug use is called "trigger reactivity."[2] The combination of individualized triggers with individualized trigger reactivity creates thousands of combinations that need to be explored to maximize a patient's resiliency against relapse.

At times, triggers induce brain activity and never enter the patient's conscious perception.[3] Early research suggests that a few addiction medications (e.g., baclofen[4]) may decrease the limbic activation created by these subliminal (unrecognized) drug triggers. We have all heard stories from addicted individuals who are surprised to learn that they have relapsed, after the fact! Self-research, exploring the vast array of one's triggers moves as many of them from the unconscious (controlled by AddictBrain) to the conscious mind (controlled by RecoveryMind). Once the patient is conscious, he or she can then develop specific trigger management skills. When an unconscious event is moved into the conscious space, it is more likely to be noticed when it recurs. If a previously practiced skill is present, this skill handles the trigger and the probability of relapse decreases.

Over the course of an addiction illness, a single patient may be sensitized to hundreds or even thousands of triggers or triggers related to his or her addiction illness. In Domain F, we explore each of these triggers, hoping to identify and develop management plans for the most difficult of them. Triggers are divided into four categories:

- Environmental triggers (e.g., seeing a drug, smelling tobacco smoke, hearing addiction-related music).
- Visceral events (body sensations, taste, or smell)
- Emotional events (a feeling that the person with an alcohol use disorder "used to drink over").
- Memory tapes (scenes that play in the mind, especially those with strong visual "tapes").

Triggers related to past using events are "conditioned"—even nonaddicted individuals are conditioned by food and other substances. For example, alcoholic beverages are paired with certain foods; a repeat diner in a French restaurant might order a specific wine with little thought after several past favorable meals (restaurants have learned to encourage this to improve profitability). Addiction generates deeper and more complex associations with abusable substances. When environmental triggers are discussed, the most common description is "external conditioned triggers." Such triggers are outside of the individual and thus external. They are conditioned, meaning the brain is entrained to expect a using event following the external stimulus. This process is known as *operant conditioning*.[5]

Added to easily identifiable external triggers are three internal processes. They are visceral (i.e., in the body) events, emotional experiences, and complex memory tapes regarding past use events.[6] Patients will develop a list of each of these four types of triggers in Worksheet F1. They are reviewed and discussed in Skill Group task F1.

Identifying and Managing Cravings

RecoveryMind Training grades cravings on a five-point scale. This scale naturally leads to a graded response, from a casual acknowledgment to the response accorded a five-alarm fire. The levels are delineated as:

Level 1. A fleeting thought of engaging in addiction that lasts less than a minute and disappears without any response on the person's part.

Level 2. A brief thought accompanied by an urge or addiction hunger lasting any period that disappears when the patient consciously focuses on another subject or physically changes his or her activity.

Level 3. A craving like that in Level 2 but one that lasts for multiple minutes and requires repeated adjustment of thinking, and/or physical relocation, or external support to abort the thoughts and urges.

Level 4. Any craving where the individual contemplates using and/or considers the presumptive benefits of using for more than ten seconds. Level 4 cravings may last for an extended period and begin to have a quality of inevitability (meaning they distort thinking to the point that the patient begins to believe the only way the cravings will go away is to use).

Level 5. Any craving that results in drug seeking or procurement in any manner.

If we ask a client to pay closer attention to craving, we are by inference obligated to teach him or her an effective management paradigm. RecoveryMind Training outlines simple responses a recovering individual can use to manage craving and improve his or her subsequent reactivity to them. The craving management process appears below.

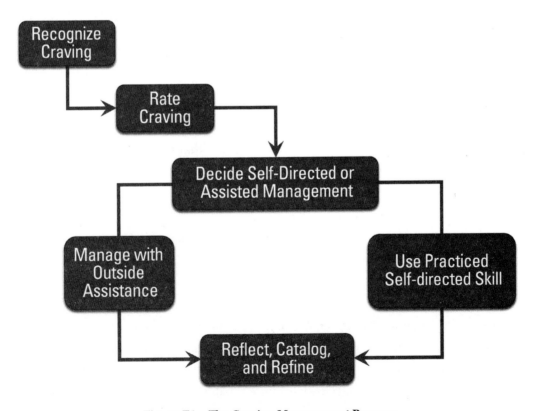

Figure F1 – The Craving Management Process

When an event is recognized as a craving, several steps need to be taken to manage that craving effectively and to prevent it from resulting in relapse. First, the patient needs to recognize that a craving has indeed occurred. If a specific trigger can be identified immediately, one should do so. If it is not immediately apparent, such research is best put off until later. Second, the individual should rate the craving using the RecoveryMind rating scale. Early in recovery, cravings at Level 2 and 3 can prove pesky at best and risky at worst. Third, patients should determine if they possess sufficient skills to manage the craving with self-skills or whether they need external support. This is often a tricky decision and one that, made incorrectly, can have devastating effects. Lower intensity cravings may be managed by simple self-directed skills. More intense cravings may require external help and support. In early recovery, clients should practice asking for assistance in managing cravings, even if they believe the intensity of the craving is not severe. Practicing self-directed craving management and asking for assistance in handling a craving are independent and mutually beneficial skills.

Individual Management

Once the patient has recognized a craving, judged its severity, and determined whether outside help is needed, craving management skills come into play. Because most individuals with substance use disorders have frequent and unpredictable cravings, it is often impractical to pull in reinforcements every time. If a client has assessed that a craving can be managed without external help, he or she should immediately respond with a craving management skill. The simple skills are:

- **Thought Blocking:** Stating with an internal voice (or, better yet, say aloud), "I am not going to think about that."
- **Thought Switching:** The individual with a substance use disorder states (internally or even better, speak out loud, "I will not think about that now; instead I will think about . . .") Thought switching can often involve a current task, a past pleasant healthy memory, a book or movie, or a past conversation. The more the individual focuses on the detail in a switched thought, the more effective the response.
- **Physical Movement:** The brain is a contextual, place-sensitive organ. Changing sensory input by movement and changing location, even a small amount, will reduce craving. Walking into another room, going outside for a moment, or getting up from a chair can abort craving.
- **Labeling the Craving as Just a Craving:** Here the individual states to him- or herself using dialog (internal or external), "Ah hah! That is a craving; nothing more." The use of language is important here. The most effective language is that of labeling ("That is a craving") rather than acknowledging its pull ("I am having a terrible craving).

More advanced skills are:

- **Reiterating that cravings come and go** if they are left alone. In the Urge Surfing Skills Group, patients learned that cravings come and go. Before they begin treatment, most people with addiction have a distorted perception that urges, especially strong ones, will persist and even continue to escalate unless they respond by using substances or engaging in addiction behaviors. After practicing Urge Surfing, patients realize that the sense of inevitability is simply a distortion produced by addiction cravings. When a craving occurs, the patient recalls the experience in Skills Group and his urge de-escalates.
- **Thinking the craving to its complete conclusion** is a "what if" process. The patient uses a narrative like the following.
  If I react to this craving by using, I will try to smoke a little heroin just to get that fuzzy warm blanket feeling. That will be followed by a hunger to use again. Over several days, I will fall into a continuous rut of using until I become hopelessly dependent. My girlfriend will know I relapsed, and this time she will kick me out for good. I will have nowhere to go. My life will fall apart. I will most likely continue to use until I overdose and die.

  The train of thought of an individual with a substance use disorder might be:
  I want to drink. The last time I drank, I was very cruel to my wife and children. This is what alcohol is doing to me. If I drink, I will lose my family. This craving will lead to an inevitable painful loss if I act on it. I know my pattern. I know where this winds up. What else could I do right now instead of ruining my life by drinking?

Such a narrative makes sure the individual in recovery aborts the fantasy of successful use, following the predictable sequence of events to its logical conclusion. I call this "putting the caboose on the train of thought."[7] AddictBrain tries to abort using thoughts at a false reward, ending at the fantasy and ignoring the long-term consequences.

Gathering External Support

If a craving is judged as intense or unpredictable or if assistance is readily available, a person in recovery is best served by asking for help. I have noticed over the years that many patients report feeling silly or weak when they ask for help. This alone can dissuade them from effective cravings management. Therefore, one of the first skills to learn in relapse prevention is how to ask for the assistance of others without falling into negative self-talk. This skill was addressed in Domain E. It is revisited here. The list of interpersonal craving management skills follows.

- **Labeling and Acknowledging to Another:** When a recovering individual goes through the sequence of verbalizing a craving and it is acknowledged by a support person, it is immediately diminished in severity and urgency—sometimes just saying it to someone else is enough. Support personnel should be trained to respond by saying, "What can I do to help?" Such a question allows the recovering individual time to reevaluate its severity, forcing him or her to consider his or her options. The support person should avoid immediately moving into fix-it mode. Quite often, the recovering person will notice the craving diminished dramatically the minute it is externalized.

- **Use Individual Skills with a Coach:** The support person may start by walking through craving skills described in the Individual Management section above. The coach might follow along with individual skills, naming and reinforcing them as they are applied: thought blocking, thought switching, and talking through the craving.

- **Changing Activity or Focus:** When a person is alone and besieged with strong cravings, changing focus may be difficult ("A person with a substance use disorder, when alone, is in dangerous territory"). The coach suggests changing the focus of the conversation, the current activity and the physical location, in that order. Learning occurs when the activities are labeled explicitly, e.g., "Let's change locations, go outside for a bit, and see how you feel." Cravings appear abruptly and in a seemingly random fashion. A line of conversation inadvertently trips up an urge. Sometimes a particular place, song, or even smell triggers a craving. When labeled and externalized, the person in recovery and his or her support person eliminate the stimulus together, increasing confidence and decreasing the probability of future relapse. One additional benefit occurs—the recovering individual experiences a deeper connection with others.

- **Controlled Trigger Exposure without Using:** A trained clinician or perceptive sponsor can also help the recovering individual extinguish the automatic craving response. I will cover this skill later in this chapter.

The RecoveryMind Relapse Prevention Model

Patients may describe a relapse as "just happening to them." One patient, when asked about his relapse, said, "I just found myself in a bar with a drink in my hand!" Such a patient is begging to be led through the relapse process, looking at the antecedents to arriving in that bar, and thought patterns that preceded them heading to that bar; these events were the *real* relapse.

RMT relapse prevention system is built upon the evidence-based relapse prevention research of Marlatt and his colleagues at the University of Washington.[8–10] Using cognitive-behavioral strategies almost thirty years ago, Dr. Marlatt developed a lucid and practical relapse model. This model has undergone extensive revision since that time;[9] one notable change in his research has modified this model to mindfulness training.[11, 12] Staff should be familiar with these reference works. A version of this model, adapted to RecoveryMind Training, appears below.

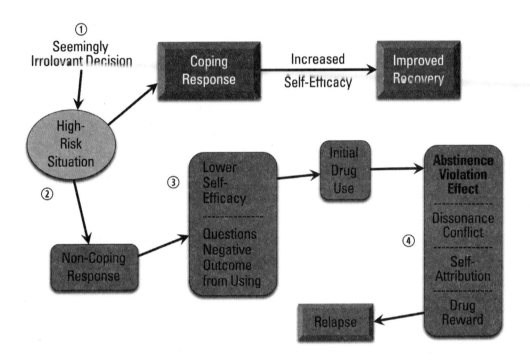

Figure F2 – Marlatt's Model of Relapse Prevention (modified from the original)

Here is a brief review of the modified Marlatt diagram. To begin, look at the upper left-hand corner. There you will see the words Seemingly Irrelevant Decision (SID). Although this concept is critical to this model, it may be difficult for patients to understand a Seemingly Irrelevant Decision and how it places them in a high-risk situation. A SID is a minor thought or decision that produces a cascade of troublesome events. For example, one day while on the way to work, a recovering individual may impulsively decide to drive a different route. Not thinking, she turns left at a traffic light thinking she is taking the indirect route to work. Suddenly, she realizes she is driving past the house of a using friend (or a bar where she used to drink). This triggers intense craving and memories of her using past. What looks like a seemingly irrelevant, almost random, decision has placed the client in a high-risk situation. Using the language of RecoveryMind Training, it can be seen that AddictBrain put what seemed to be an irrelevant thought in the client's head, knowing it could lead to relapse. SIDs are easy enough to understand in the abstract. If a patient is well along the way of internalizing the concepts of RecoveryMind Training, such an analysis may at times be intuitively recognizable. On the other hand, note that SIDs are much easier to identify retrospectively. Asking individuals to identify a SID proactively can challenge them. How to encourage self-examination is to encourage the recovering individual to be skeptical of his or her own thoughts. Said another way, "Don't always believe what you think" is a maxim that applies to early recovery.

The next inflection point along the path to relapse is the High-Risk Situation. A high-risk situation is a social, geographical, emotional, or interpersonal circumstance where the recovering individual is at an increased relapse risk. Relapse prevention training teaches the individual to notice and act as soon as possible to mitigate such situations. Once trained, the recovering individual goes on alert in such circumstances, recognizing danger and the possibility of relapse. High-risk situations happen nearly every day when one is early in recovery.

Figure F2 illustrates how any high-risk situation is a crossroads. A coping response occurs when clients make the right choice in such a circumstance. A coping response almost always involves action. When the right path is taken, they develop an increased sense of self-efficacy—the path at the top of the diagram. They have taken a step to harden their recovery by experiencing the benefits in the path taken.

A brief discussion about self-efficacy in needed here. The concept of self-efficacy is sometimes difficult for therapists who use twelve-step principles. Self-efficacy is different from "taking back control." The concept of self-efficacy has elements of self-esteem, combined with an ability to make healthy choices. When clients respond to a high-risk situation with a coping response and observes themselves muster multiple resources to subvert AddictBrain's agenda, their sense of helplessness abates. These resources include previous relapse prevention training, the advice of one's sponsor and often a higher power. This is a fine balance, however. Danger can sneak in the back door when a recovering person asserts, "I outwitted that danger, and this makes me stronger. Next time, I will be able to go to that party and stay all night without using."

On the other hand, each coping response improves one's recovery program. Increased self-esteem and the sense that recovery is an attainable goal are balanced with a healthy respect for the illness. When AddictBrain has been thwarted once or twice, some individuals confuse these short-term successes with hardened armor against all future relapse. During relapse prevention training, it is important to congratulate each coping response and at the same time prevent the recovering individual from falling into the fantasy of impenetrable protection from relapse.

Now follow Figure F2 down the other branch. If the recovering person fails to make a coping response, he or she begins a cascade of events that build on each other, each increasing the probability of relapse. If the individual fails to make a coping response, a series of internal states emerge. His or her self-esteem decreases and helplessness increases. AddictBrain whispers, "You know you're going to use." The recovering individual contemplates the possibility of a good outcome from substance use, despite overwhelming evidence to the contrary.

The moment the first use occurs, a cascade of events befalls the recovering individual. Marlatt labeled this cascade the Abstinence Violation Effect (AVE). I have slightly modified his original AVE in Figure F2. The first element in this cascade is Dissonance Conflict. Dissonance conflict arises when a particular belief or self-concept is contradicted by current actions or behaviors.[13] The conflict produces significant emotional distress. The distress most often fuels the relapse rather than interrupt it. The second component of AVE is self-attribution. The likelihood of a continuation of the relapse process is increased by how strongly the individual attributed the breach to fixed personal attributes ("I have no willpower") rather than controllable causes ("I should have used better coping skills in this situation").[14, 15] Self-attribution leads to a further sense of hopelessness and defectiveness—prominent characteristics in the victims of addiction disorders.[15]

To Marlatt's original model, I add an important biological component of relapse. Once an addictive substance or behavior is introduced into the brain, reward pathways dramatically increase the probability of continued use. This phenomenon, drug reward that comes from first use, adds to the prior two components of the abstinence violation effect. The combination of dissonance conflict, self-attribution and reinforced craving unleash a mighty storm of relapse. Continued substance use or addiction behaviors seem inevitable and a full-blown relapse ensues.

Interventions to Prevent Relapse

Referring to Figure F1, recall labels ① through ④ in the diagram. Each of these refers to specific points along the relapse prevention model where interventions prove effective.

Point ① – Seemingly Irrelevant Decisions

The first point of intervention is noted to occur during the process of Seemingly Irrelevant Decisions. Even though this is the first and most effective point of intervention, it is the most difficult for individuals to recognize before the fact, especially in early recovery. Seemingly irrelevant decisions are by their very nature *seemingly irrelevant*. Recognizing what appears to be a benign and inconsequential choice as a dangerous path to relapse requires practiced self-reflection. Some patients may never be able to proactively recognize a SID.

The best way to open the door to SID recognition is by teaching curiosity about self, combined with a touch of self-doubt. Such curiosity is acquired through work in Domain D (with the assistance of Skills Group D3 and Worksheet D6 discussed in Assignment Group D4). Early in recovery, the client should weigh each decision to determine if it is "In the service of AddictBrain or RecoveryMind."[16] Clients should be taught to question their decisions frequently, setting aside judgments of right or wrong. An individual who has learned to recognize his or her own SIDs will describe these destructive decisions as spontaneously popping up in his or her thoughts, arising out of nowhere. Impulsivity is rampant in addiction and early recovery. The antidote is curiosity and self-examination. Self-examination often identifies SIDs with a slow, burning realization that a contemplated action is promoting relapse, not sustaining recovery.

Patients will have an easier time listing past high-risk situations, especially those that led to relapse. The therapist acknowledges this recognition as valuable and follows this up with an important question: "What were the ideas, emotions, external pressures, and decisions that got you to that high-risk situation?" Such work leads to the exploration of seemingly irrelevant decisions and a deeper commitment to discovering SIDs as part of a robust relapse prevention strategy.

Point ② – High-Risk Situations

In RMT's relapse prevention training, the most time is spent identifying high-risk situations and developing specific response plans for the most likely circumstances. To determine how to manage such events, RecoveryMind Training divides high-risk situations into three categories:

- **Address Now:** These high-risk situations are part of everyday life. The recovering individual must acquire skills to manage such situations immediately.
- **Delay Exposure:** Certain high-risk situations should initially be avoided until the patient learns specific skills to manage the given situation. Such circumstances often require unpracticed skills to avoid relapse. These high-risk situations represent events that must eventually be faced to avoid an overly restrictive life in recovery.
- **Avoid Forever:** Circumstances labeled Avoid Forever are extremely dangerous. Such situations commonly offer no value to the recovering individual. Many of these situations are simply a relapse waiting to happen. Recovering individuals often expose themselves to this type of high-risk situation out of false confidence or a foolish need to "prove they are strong in recovery."

Table F1 provides examples of each of the three types of high-risk situations dividing them up into one of these three categories.

Table F1: Examples of High-Risk Situation Examples

Example of a high-risk situation	Type	Comments
Entering a bar for any reason unless to transit to a restaurant.	Delay Exposure	In the first several years of recovery, should be completely avoided. Later, anything more than a brief stint in a bar should be avoided or treated with extreme caution. It may be necessary in the future if there is a reason the client should be there (e.g., waiting for a dinner table).
Meeting up with acquaintances the client used with in the past.	Delay Exposure	This varies depending on the role a friend had in the patient's life. Patients will commonly underestimate how dangerous past using friends are to their recovery.
Getting in an argument with your spouse.	Address Now	Interpersonal conflict is unavoidable. Instead of avoiding conflict, patients should be taught interpersonal effectiveness.
Sitting in front of a pile of cocaine.	Avoid Forever	Some addicts think it a sign of bravery and bravado to continue to expose themselves to alcohol and other drugs. This is just foolhardy.
Driving past a favorite bar enroute elsewhere.	Delay Exposure	Find a different route to avoid driving past the bar at first. Later, desensitize the experience with sponsor or recovery coach.
Having excess money in a pocket or purse.	Delay Exposure	This is especially true for individuals who have purchased drugs with cash.
Dealing with painful feelings related to addiction.	Address Now	Recovery is filled with painful emotions. If appropriate, such issues should be addressed in Domain C.
Watching movies with explicit alcohol or other drug use or drug dealing.	Delay Exposure	The exact process of desensitization regarding explicit movies varies from individual to individual. Movies that glorify alcohol or drug use are the most problematic; however, even negative portrayals can trigger cravings.
Placing work or social obligations over recovery.	Avoid Forever	Depending on the severity of addiction, individuals must learn how much emphasis needs to be placed on recovery over work, home, and social obligations. The tricky part of this distinction is how much emphasis. Obviously, this changes over time; early in recovery, work and social obligations need to take a back seat consistently.
Attending a party where the primary goal is alcohol or other drug intoxication.	Avoid Forever	Patients should be taught how to assess which social situations are safe and which are problematic. Social situations where intoxication is the primary goal are always unsafe and will be boring to the recovering individual.

Example of a high-risk situation	Type	Comments
Attend a work event where alcohol will be served	Delay Exposure	The social use of alcohol is prevalent in many work environments. Individuals who work around or entertain with alcohol need specific alcohol refusal training.
Airplane travel or boat cruise where alcohol is freely served and encouraged.	Delay Exposure	Individuals whose work includes frequent airline travel have heavy alcohol exposure. Ship cruises expose travelers to alcohol almost continuously. Specific relapse prevention strategies should be practiced before engaging in these activities.
Overcoming social anxiety in order to attend therapy or support groups.	Address Now	Social support is a large part of the recovery process. Individuals who have social anxieties need specific training to help realize the benefits of the many recovery offerings that occur in a group format.
Going to a musical concert where alcohol or other drugs are used socially.	Delay Exposure	Musical concerts of all genres are associated with alcohol or other drug use. An individual in early recovery should delay such exposure. When the time is right to attend, he or she should attend with others in recovery, helping each other control their immediate environment.
Attending a family function where alcohol is served.	Delay Exposure	Family functions with alcohol are a double whammy, since easy access to alcohol is combined with the inevitable emotional content of such situations.
Staying alone in a hotel or motel with a "minibar."	Delay Exposure	Many hotels with minibars have keys. When checking in, the recovering individual can refuse the key or ask for a room without this unneeded temptation.
Volunteering in a shelter that houses actively using drug addicts.	Delay Exposure	Working in a volunteer capacity helps the recovering person gain self-esteem and increases gratitude and interpersonal connection. However, depending on his or her personality structure, such jobs can create additional risks. It is best to review these decisions with a sponsor or therapist.
Spending long periods of time alone and away from recovery support.	Delay Exposure	Recovery is a daily process that erodes when is not properly maintained. A recovering individual should have consistent contact with his or her recovering community early in his or her journey. Prolonged periods away from recovery support should be carefully considered.
Traveling to locations where support group meetings are unavailable.	Delay Exposure	As with the situation above, individuals who must travel away from their support network should find alternative means of buttressing their recovery.

Worksheet F3 helps patients catalog high-risk situations. Skill building around the more complex and unavoidable high-risk situations occurs in Skills Group F3.

Point ③ – After Non-Coping Response

Interrupting the process of relapse becomes increasingly more difficult as one proceeds down the road toward relapse. This does not mean, however, that relapse is inevitable. Aborting the relapse process at Point ③ starts by recognizing that things have progressed to this dangerous point. Curiosity combined with a previous understanding of this stage in the relapse prevention model is potent medicine. The recovering individual should be taught to recognize and retroflect when a drop in self-efficacy occurs, "Why am I feeling so vulnerable at this very moment?" Certain thought patterns are extremely dangerous to the recovering individual—Alcoholics Anonymous calls these thoughts "stinking thinking." The recovering individual should ring an internal alarm bell during the most dangerous of these moments. A common example is Point ③, when this subversive idea emerges: "just this once using alcohol or other drugs might be a good idea." If the thought is coupled with the additional notion that substance use will have no negative consequences, the fantasy becomes an especially dangerous delusion.

If a recovering individual unwittingly exposes him- or herself to a high-risk situation and then falls into Point ③ in this relapse model, immediate action is needed. The individual should physically move away from the high-risk situation ("put your wallet back in your pocket, step away from the bar, and walk out the door"). Next, support troops should be enlisted. When the individual in this circumstance establishes connection with a sponsor or other support group members, he is halfway out of the woods. The sponsor is called, a simple instruction to immediately exit from the high-risk situation is issued, and he executes a relapse prevention behavior. Each successive execution of a healthy reaction reinforces future coping responses and stabilizes recovery.

Point ④ – Abstinence Violation Effect

Moving along the process of relapse, we come to the Point ④ in my model, the Abstinence Violation Effect. Patients who have been traumatized by previous relapse understand fully the pain that occurs immediately after the first sip of alcohol or experience using their drug of choice. A whole cascade of events occurs. The most common and unfortunate result is a fury of thoughts and behaviors that comprise the Abstinence Violation Effect, and the relapse process is complete. Nonetheless, some individuals can abort relapse here, surviving the maelstrom of the AVE.

The techniques for aborting full relapse at Point ④ are like those at Point ③. Let's walk through specific responses to each of the elements of the AVE with Anthony. Assume Anthony attends a sports event with his previous drinking buddies (a high-risk situation). He starts thinking he could have a few drinks with his friends without consequences (Point ③—Questions negative outcome from using). Impulsively, he picks up a beer, drinking half of it quickly (Point ④—Abstinence Violation Effect). His mind is quickly flooded by the AVE. His brain generates dissonance conflict. ("You told everyone, including yourself that you are in recovery and here you are drinking a beer!"). Anthony pronounces his recovery a failure and, by extension, he is a failure. This is self-attribution, another element of the AVE. These thoughts and feelings combine with the initial effect of alcohol, which dulls the pain and promotes continued alcohol use. This is the third part of the AVE—rewarding effects of the drug.

To pull out of the relapse process, a client needs to correct his thinking, *Relapse is unfortunate but does occur in recovery, I can see this as a setback but a learning experience,* and *I made a bad decision being around my old drinking friends, it is a bad decision in an otherwise good recovery.* The client needs to make dramatic changes in his environment. Flee the sports event with any kind of excuse, call a friend in recovery immediately, and seek out others in recovery, such as a sponsor and a recovery support group.

As you can see, relapse prevention becomes more difficult as one moves from Point ① to Point ④. As one moves further down the line, cognitive distortion increases. Small quantities of addicting substances radically alter goal-oriented behavior, moving from recovery goals to the goals of AddictBrain. Process-oriented relapse prevention is complex and is rarely helpful without the procedural learning that comes from role-play. This is discussed further in Skills Group F3.

Therapeutic Elements in Domain F

Domain F has three Skills Groups:

F1) Asking and Providing Help with Cravings

F2) Learning to Surf the Urge

F3) High-Risk Situation Role Play

There are four Assignment Group tasks in Domain F:

F1) Review of the **Triggers** Worksheet F1

F2) Review of the **Cravings Management** Worksheet F2

F3) Initial review of the **High-risk Situation** Worksheet F3

F4) Second review of the **High-Risk Situation** Worksheet F3

There are four Worksheets in Domain F:

F1) The **Triggers** Worksheet

F2) The **Cravings Management** Worksheet

F3) The **High-Risk Situation** Worksheet

F4) The **Emotions and Relapse** Worksheet. This worksheet explores the interplay between specific emotions and drug use or addiction behaviors.

Domain F: Skills Groups

Skills Group F1: Asking and Providing Help with Cravings

This Skills Group may not take an entire hour-long session; it can be squeezed in when a half hour is available. The skill is simple in principle: asking someone else for help managing cravings. Many people with substance use disorders find it more difficult in actual practice.

The leader asks two group members to sit facing one another for the initial demonstration. The protagonist thinks of an image, thought, or emotion that will induce a craving. They sit quietly entertaining that trigger. After a moment, the protagonist looks at his or her partner and asks for help with a craving he or she is experiencing. The partner responds with affirmation, "I will help you with this craving. What would you like from me?"

Skills Group F2: Surfing the Urge

This Skills Group is nearly identical to a skill learned in Domain Skills Group C2, Surfing Uncomfortable Emotions. This process was first described by Dr. Alan Marlatt.[17] The group begins with a brief introductory lecture. In this lecture, the leader reiterates characteristics of cravings or urges. Cravings are described as a normal response in the addicted brain. Participants are discouraged from self-judgment regarding cravings. Several thought distortions about cravings are emphasized. First, when cravings appear, they have a quality of urgency. By surfing the urge, allowing it to do well without acting on it, watching it rise and fall and by preventing a behavioral response, urges become more manageable. Stronger cravings have a quality of inevitability. This means that the victim of such cravings feels as if the only way to make the craving go away is to give in to it. These are distortions created by these urges. They can be overcome by practicing the skill called Surfing the Urge. The last element in this brief introductory lecture is a warning. Patients are not to practice this skill unless they are in a safe environment for a sustained period after this exercise.

Next, patients are instructed to sit quietly and focus inward. The instructor leads the group in a brief meditative practice. Participants are then asked to recall a past urge or past using event that was powerful. Returning to the meditative state, each participant asks the urge to return. They are instructed to remain in the room, watching the hunger rise and fall. Participants may notice that only part of their stream of consciousness is occupied by the craving. They are instructed to notice the qualities of the craving. Does it have a taste or smell? Does it make them want to move? Is there an ache or pain associated with it? Which specific emotions arise alongside it? Such questions create distance between the craving and the experience of it. If the craving briefly goes away, participants are encouraged to sit quietly and watch when it does return.

Especially important in this process are recognizing the rise and fall of the intensity of the craving, its relative urgency, and the qualities of that urgency (urgency often creates physical movement). After a moment, participants are encouraged to recall a calm river or stream. In their mind's eye, they construct a small raft and place the craving on it. In their mind's eye they gently push the raft containing the craving into the current and watch it slowly float downstream. This is followed by periods of centering breath work, slowly opening their eyes, and returning to the room.

The leader then encourages discussion. If a participant derails into self-destructive drug romancing, this is labeled as such and stopped. Participants are encouraged to rely on the support of each other throughout the day. Such support does not include asking for lurid details about each other's craving experiences. Rather, participants check in with each other to ensure they are safe and committed to ongoing treatment.

Skills Group F3: High-Risk Situation Role-Play

This Skills Group begins with a protagonist reading his high-risk situation. The director or leader selects a high-risk situation well adapted to role-playing. At times, the protagonist's brief description is read aloud several times, allowing for feedback and questioning by the audience. When everyone has a clear image of this high-risk situation, role-play begins.

The identified protagonist goes center stage, describing the scene in as much detail as possible. Auxiliaries and props are brought into the scene to augment its symbolic reality. The protagonist is encouraged to describe what he is experiencing, especially focused on the voices in his head. One common conflicting voice arises is a critical controlling voice ("What were you thinking allowing yourself to get into this situation?"). A second, nearly universal, internal voice is that of cajoling AddictBrain ("It's good hanging out with your old using friends, they really get you"). Auxiliaries are enrolled to play these and any other internal dialogue that emerges through the scene.

Using doubling and mirroring, the protagonist experiences this high-risk situation in its entirety. At times, these high-risk situations lead to early childhood wounding. If appropriately trained, the leader may choose to follow a more traditional psychodrama process and work toward catharsis of this past trauma. More commonly, the protagonist and members of the audience build a repertoire of strengthening reactions to this high-risk situation. If the protagonist is stuck, he can pull in auxiliary helpers who suggest healthy coping responses. The leader carefully weighs the protagonist's reaction to any suggestions, giving him wide latitude in rejecting and refining suggestions until he feels just right. Several coping responses are practiced repeatedly and with increasing refinement until they have the potential to become automatic when faced with this high-risk situation.

When this protagonist's scene comes to its conclusion, auxiliaries disenrolled and all members return to the circle. Critique of the previous scene is discouraged. Instead, members of the group describe reactions to the role-play, how it might apply to them, and what was felt while watching the work. If time allows, a second protagonist is chosen, and the cycle repeats. This Skills Group may extend over multiple sessions—it is foundational and critical procedural learning in RecoveryMind Training.

The protagonist then suggests one of several approaches, for example:
- Let's try talking about something else.
- Let me describe the craving, and I will talk it through relapse and my eventual downfall.
- Will you walk around the room or go outside with me for a moment?
- I would like to sit together and try mindfulness meditation with you.
- I would like to talk about the painful feelings that trigger this craving.

The protagonist's helper agrees, and the first technique is practiced. The protagonist then reflects on the help or lack of help that the technique offered in ameliorating the craving. A second and third technique may be asked for and practiced. The helper then provides feedback. The roles are switched and the exercise repeats.

Once the demonstration is complete, the leader asks for questions. A brief discussion ensues. The group breaks up into dyads and each couple practice both sides, asking for help and providing help. The skills practiced in this exercise are learning to recognize what a craving feels like, learning to ask for help, practicing craving management, and learning to help others. Some participants may see this exercise as easy; others may find it very difficult. Overly self-reliant participants may be especially troubled by this group.

Domain F: Assignment Groups Tasks

Assignment Group Task F1

During this Assignment Group task, the patient reads the contents of the Triggers Worksheet. Group members ask questions about the triggers and, in doing so, clarify the definition of a trigger for all group members. Discussions about the effects of the trigger on the protagonist are helpful, preparing them for future assignments. Members may suggest other triggers to help build a robust list ("I get triggered when I hear someone flicking a lighter, does this trigger you?").

Assignment Group Task F2

For this Assignment Group, clients bring their Cravings Management Worksheet F2 to group for review and discussion. Each protagonist goes through his or her list describing each craving. Group members or the protagonist themselves may be triggered by simply reading, describing, or discussing a craving, especially if it is universal. This can often be a helpful moment to practice cravings management with the group at-large. Cravings are the same for many people, some are universal—the ones that are universal are exploited by advertising agencies. The leader balances completing the assignment with helpful experience in managing cravings.

One important concept from RecoveryMind Training is helpful here. The concept is the difference between talking about a craving and inducing euphoric recall. Discussing cravings helps patients understand and normalize them. It provides a limited dose exposure to a craving without a subsequent relapse. Such discussion slowly extinguishes the intensity of the craving through repeated exposure.

However, discussions about cravings tend to deteriorate into euphoric recall. The transition from helpful discussion to euphoric recall is subtle and varies from person to person. Once in the mode of euphoric recall, the discussant displays increasing positive affect, a pressure to his speech, possible fidgetiness or agitation, and a strong desire to continue the current subject. Skilled leaders learn to detect this subtle transition and interrupt euphoric recall before it becomes destructive. One helpful technique is to stop the discussion and focus on group feeling and process. The question, "What is everyone feeling right now?" is followed by "How does this feel different than the group felt just five minutes ago?" When group members can identify the difference, the leader goes on to describe euphoric recall and the need to avoid such recall. Patients further along in the recovery process are much more skilled at distinguishing euphoric recall from healthy discussions of cravings management.

In going over the craving list, the protagonist describes the qualities of selected cravings using the following list:

- **U** – Urgency (when it comes you have a strong feeling like you must use—now)
- **I** – Intensity (when this craving comes, it is intense)
- **D** – Has a long duration (lasts a long time)
- **R** – Recurrence (feels like it will come back, over and over)
- **P** – Is persistent (remains despite efforts to push it away)

During the discussion of craving qualities, the group often seeks to clarify the meaning of each of the quality terms. Note that the primary goal of elucidating the qualities of a craving is to produce a certain amount of intellectual distance and emotional acceptance of the craving state. Understanding all of the subtle nuances of a given craving had no validated benefit.

Finally, the protagonist rates the relative risk or danger of cravings. Other group members might provide feedback about the danger inherent in certain craving states.

Assignment Group Task F3

During this group task, clients bring High-Risk Situation Worksheet F3 to group for initial review. Each reads his or her list of high-risk situations. The group provides feedback, asks for details, and encourages the protagonist to think about other situations ("David, I remember you talking about how your brother-in-law comes to visit several times a year. He brings several fifths of alcohol and pot with him and spends most of the time getting high when he is in your house. This is surely a high-risk situation.") If the list is insufficient or superficial, the protagonist is encouraged to dig deeper and bring it back for a second review.

If the list is complete and comprehensive, the protagonist reads the list again suggesting categories for each situation using this list:

- **N** – Address now.
- **D** – Delay exposure to this situation until later. The patient will return to situations in this category in order to extinguish the cravings and help him or her lead a less restricted life in recovery.
- **A** – Always avoid. Items in this category are extremely dangerous situations for clients. This would include direct exposure to using friends or drugs or to being in an unhealthy situation in which the client repeatedly relapsed in the past.

The protagonist discusses the situations with the group, searching for healthy management plans.

The protagonist, David suggests, "I will just not sit with him when he is drinking in my house." The group says, "Whoa, that is not enough," and follows it up with "Tell your sister and brother-in-law that they cannot come and visit for the next several months. This will buy you time. When you feel stronger, get on the phone with them and let them know they are welcome to visit, but if they are staying in your apartment, they cannot be using anything during the visit. If that is too tough for them, suggest they stay in a hotel. You will then have to limit the time you spend with them."

The leader will tend to direct this group, offering critique and management plans they know will work from experience. They should restrain themselves, however. When other group members think through other's dilemmas, they empower their own plans and actions. If a weak management plan is suggested, the leader says, "What do other people think about this plan? What are its strengths and weaknesses?"

Assignment Group Task F4

In this Group Task, patients bring their High-Risk Situation Worksheet F3 to group for a second review. The second time around, the protagonist and group members focus on the Management Plan for each High-Risk Situation. Is the selected category correct? Which management plans are the most difficult? Which high-risk situations have the most risk (and therefore need the most practice)? The protagonist and the group discuss the list on Worksheet F3, suggesting one or more situations to role-play in Skills Group F3.

Domain F: Relapse Prevention Worksheets

Overview of Worksheets

In many ways, Domain F Relapse Prevention is the most important area of treatment. Patients need to learn relapse prevention skills to the highest level of fidelity to achieve long-term recovery. For this reason, I encourage staff to gently push patients when completing these worksheets.

Work in relapse prevention requires a patient who has sufficient insight into his illness and a willingness to sit with disquieting feelings that emerge when working in this area. For these reasons, Domain F is the last of the six domains. Many times, a patient will wait until he has months in recovery before deep work in Domain F is addressed.

There are four Worksheets in Domain F:
- F1) The **Triggers** Worksheet. This Worksheet helps patients categorize the myriad triggers or triggers that stimulate craving or relapse. Once this worksheet is complete, it is reviewed in an Assignment Group.
- F2) The **Cravings Management** Worksheet. The Cravings Management Worksheet follows seamlessly from the Triggers Worksheet. Patients explore their cravings in this worksheet. They then carry it to Assignment Group for discussion.
- F3) The **High-Risk Situation** Worksheet. The High-Risk Situation Worksheet is the longest and most complex worksheet in Domain F. The patient fills Column One and then brings his or her worksheet to the Assignment Group. The Assignment Group should thoroughly investigate the list of high-risk situations and ensure they are complete. The patient then finishes this worksheet and returns to the Assignment Group for additional suggestions and feedback.
- F4) The **Emotions and Relapse** Worksheet. This worksheet explores the interplay between specific emotions and drug use or addiction behaviors.

Worksheet F1: Triggers Worksheet

RecoveryMind Training defines triggers as the earliest point in the relapse process. The most common sequence that occurs is:

$$\text{Trigger} \Rightarrow \text{Craving} \Rightarrow \text{High-Risk Situation} \Rightarrow \text{Relapse}$$

Note that this sequence does not always present or escalate in this simple sequence. However, it is always easiest to get off the road to relapse at the trigger stage. The earlier you derail the process of relapse, the higher the likelihood of continued success.

A trigger is something that occurs outside and/or within you that induces craving or relapse. They can be thoughts, sensations, emotions, recalled scenes, images, or other visual events and memories. They can be smells or tastes, single sounds or music. In completing this worksheet, the client should carefully recall failed attempts to decrease or stop using, looking for the initial trigger that prompted relapse or continued use. Be diligent and inquisitive. You may be surprised by the number and type of triggers you discover. Go over the list with peers and family. They might have suggestions to add to your list.

First, write down your list of triggers in column ①. When you list a feeling or an emotional event that triggers you, be as specific as possible (e.g., that dark, angry feeling I have about myself when I repeatedly disappoint my son).

Go back through the list and in the column ②, categorize your triggers according to this classification:
- **T** – Thought
- **E** – Event
- **B** – Body sensations, taste, smells
- **F** – Feelings (be specific)
- **M** – Memories that cause you to cringe or trigger you when they play out in your head

In column ③, rate how troublesome this trigger is to you. Rate your triggers on a list of 1 to 5. A score of 1 would indicate the trigger was irritating but not dangerous. A score of 5 would be a trigger that would put you at very high risk of relapse or induce a craving that would seem intolerable (and therefore put you at high risk for relapse).

Describe the Trigger or Triggers ①	Type ②	Relative Risk (1–5) ③

① Describe the Trigger or Triggers	② Type	③ Relative Risk (1–5)

Worksheet F2: Cravings Management

Cravings are internal sensations that plague everyone in recovery. Cravings are a normal, biological response created by addiction. They often get stronger and more persistent after an individual stops using. Paradoxically, they may be stronger or more frequent during times when the client feels the strongest commitment to quit. Cravings are AddictBrain fighting back. Whatever you do, do not judge your recovery based upon the frequency or intensity of your cravings. Some people try to suppress cravings. This too is a mistake. When you learn to recognize all your cravings, even the subtlest ones, you will be best equipped to manage them.

This worksheet is designed to help you catalog the myriad cravings you experience or feel. First describe cravings that you have experienced in the past. In column ①, write down every craving you can recall. Take your time with this and search deeply to build a comprehensive list. Then set this worksheet aside for a day. Coming back to it later, write down others that have come to you. Be as thorough as you can. Next, fill column ② with the trigger or triggers that seems to promote this craving. If you cannot come up with what seems to produce a specific craving, simply leave column ② blank. Many cravings seem to appear out of nowhere. Next fill in column ③ with any of the following qualities based upon the following code system. A craving can have zero, one, or many of these qualities.

- **U**–Urgency (When it comes you have a strong feeling like you must use—now!)
- **I**–Intensity (When this craving comes, it is intense.)
- **D**–Has a long duration (Lasts a long time.)
- **R**–Recurrence (Feels like it will come back, over and over.)
- **P**–Is persistent (Remains despite efforts to push it away.)

Finally, rate each craving in your list in column ④, based upon how dangerous it is to your recovery. A 1 is mildly dangerous and a 5 is extremely dangerous.

① Describe the Craving	② Brought on by?	③ Qualities	④ Danger

① Describe the Craving	② Brought on by?	③ Qualities	④ Danger

Worksheet F3: High-Risk Situation

High-Risk Situations can occur in countless situations, all of which have one common characteristic: they place you in a situation where you must act to prevent relapse. They may be social (going to a party that you thought would be recovery safe, but when you get there you find out it is not), emotional (getting in a difficult argument with a loved one where, in the past you always wound up using), or logistical (having a drug dealer show up at your house asking for money or offering drugs). Each person has his or her own unique set of high-risk situations. Each recovering individual must plan how to successfully navigate these situations.

In column ①, list your high-risk situations. Ask for help from family, sponsor, friends, and peers in treatment. When you hear other people describing high-risk situations, consider whether a variant of that situation applies to you. When you have completed this list in column ①, STOP. Bring the list to Assignment Group, asking for time there. The group will review your list, helping you refine your list. They will also help you divide your list into one of the following categories of high-risk situations:

- **N** – Address now.
- **D** – Delay your exposure to this situation until later. You will have to return to situations in this category to extinguish the cravings and help you lead a less restricted life in recovery.
- **A** – Always avoid. Items in this category are extremely dangerous situations for you. This would include direct exposure to using friends or drugs or being in an unhealthy situations in which you repeatedly relapsed in the past.

When you have presented your initial list in Assignment Group, come back to complete this worksheet. First complete column ③ for each item. Assign each high-risk situation a risk value. A value of 1 has a mild tendency to induce relapse and a value of 5 will almost certainly result in relapse. When you have completed this, consider how this high-risk situation should be managed in the future. Your Assignment Group will have also provided you with suggestions as to a proper management plan. Note that for Category A high-risk situations, the plan is the same as the category: Always avoid. However, you should fill in column ④ with a consistent plan as to how you will always avoid this high-risk situation.

When you complete all columns, bring this worksheet back to the Assignment Group for more work. There, you will present your list again, focusing on how you will refine your management plan for the highest risk situations. You will want to role-play some of the more complex high-risk situations in the skill group dedicated to managing high-risk situations.

① High-Risk Situation	② Category	③ Relative Risk (1–5)	④ Management Plan

① High-Risk Situation	② Category	③ Relative Risk (1–5)	④ Management Plan

Worksheet F4: Emotions and Relapse

Many recovering individuals are sensitive to certain feelings. Some are not sensitive in the sense of always knowing how they feel; indeed, they often run away from disquieting emotions by suppressing feelings, acting out on them, and other human maneuvers that do anything besides simply experiencing emotions.

In this worksheet, you will examine feelings and emotional states that can lead to relapse. Sometimes the best way of finding such emotions is to scan back through your life, recalling times when you were emotionally distraught, paying attention to when a feeling state prompted using or even caused a relapse.

Write down the components of these emotional events in Column ①. Define the emotion or emotions as best you can in Column ②. Be diligent in trying to find the word or words that capture the feeling best, referring to the feeling list in Worksheet C1 for help. You may need to come back to this worksheet many times to make a comprehensive survey of emotions that are closely related to your addiction. In Column ③, enter the relative risk of experiencing this feeling state; a 1 is low risk a 5 is very high risk for relapse or continued use. If, for example, every time your husband threatens to leave because you continue to drink (Column ①), you feel abandoned and hopeless (Column ②), and you invariably drink, enter a 5 in Column ③.

① Event Around the Feeling or Emotion	② List the Emotion(s)	③ Relative Risk (1–5)

① Event Around the Feeling or Emotion	② List the Emotion(s)	③ Relative Risk (1–5)

Domain F: Progress Assessment Form

RecoveryMind Training – Relapse Prevention

Domain F Recovery Skill	Date: Patient			Staff			Date: Patient			Staff			Date: Patient			Staff		
	B	I	C	B	I	C	B	I	C	B	I	C	B	I	C	B	I	C
Understands the meaning of and difference between a Trigger, Craving, High-Risk Situation, and a Relapse.																		
Can identify and grade cravings when they occur.																		
Understands and has practiced several of the six individual craving management skills.																		
Has identified the most dangerous personal cravings and has committed an automatic response to memory.																		
Has successfully participated in Urge Surfing training.																		
Has a complete list of high-risk situations and a plan to manage each one.																		
Knows the high-risk situations to Delay Exposure and to Always Avoid. Has exhibited a commitment to this portion of relapse prevention																		
Has recognized and reviewed several past and at least one current Seemingly Irrelevant Decision(s).																		
Has a comprehensive description of the emotional states that create the highest risk for relapse and has a memorized response plan when each one occurs.																		

This evaluation is completed by both the patient or client (self-assessment) and his or her therapist or staff members on this one form. After starting work on a skill, place the approximate start date in the column provided. The patient or client fills out the form first. A therapist or staff member performs the same evaluation, placing a check mark in each row that indicates progress in assigned Recovery Skills. This process may need to be repeated several times as work progresses in each domain.

A check mark in the **B** column signifies that work has begun. The **I** column should be checked if the patient is in an intermediate or midway through his or her work on this item, and the **C** column should be checked if the patient has made sufficient progress in the skill to move forward to his or her next task. Review and discussion of this form helps patients and therapists set clear treatment expectations and recovery goals.

Domain F: Relapse Prevention Notes

1.   American Society of Addiction Medicine. "The Definition of Addiction." ASAM, http://www.asam.org/docs/public-policy-statements/1definition_of_addiction_long_4-11.pdf?sfvrsn=2.

2.   A. J. Jasinska, F. A. Stein, J. Kaiser, M. J. Naumer, and Y. Yalachkov. "Factors Modulating Neural Reactivity to Drug Cues in Addiction: A Survey of Human Neuroimaging Studies." *Neuroscience & Biobehavioral Reviews* 38, no. 0 (2014): 1–16.

3.   A. R. Childress, R. N. Ehrman, Z. Wang, Y. Li, N. Sciortino, J. Hakun, W. Jens, *et al.* "Prelude to Passion: Limbic Activation by 'Unseen' Drug and Sexual Cues." *PLoS One* 3, no. 1 (2008): e1506.

4.   K. A. Young, T. R. Franklin, D. C. Roberts, K. Jagannathan, J. J. Suh, R. R. Wetherill, Z. Wang, *et al.* "Nipping Cue Reactivity in the Bud: Baclofen Prevents Limbic Activation Elicited by Subliminal Drug Cues." *J Neurosci* 34, no. 14 (2014): 5038–43.

5.   B. F. Skinner. *Science and Human Behavior*. New York,: Macmillan, 1953.

6.   RecoveryMind Training calls these "Addiction Memory" events. They are postulated to be similar and stored in the brain in a manner similar to post traumatic stress disorder (PTSD).

7.   Thanks to Robert Weinhold, MS for this phrase.

8.   S. Bowen, N. Chawla, and G. Marlatt. *Mindfulness-Based Relapse Prevention for Addictive Behaviors: A Clinician's Guide*. Guilford Press, 2010.

9.   M. E. Larimer, R. S. Palmer, and G. A. Marlatt. "Relapse Prevention. An Overview of Marlatt's Cognitive-Behavioral Model." *Alcohol Res Health* 23, no. 2 (1999): 151–60.

10.   A. Marlatt, and D. Donovan. *Relapse Prevention, Maintenance Strategies in the Treatment of Addictive Behaviors*. Second ed.: Guilford Press, 2007.

11.   K. Witkiewitz, G. A. Marlatt, and D. Walker. "Mindfulness-Based Relapse Prevention for Alcohol and Substance Use Disorders." *Journal of Cognitive Psychotherapy* 19, no. 3 (2005): 211–28.

12.   S. Bowen, K. Witkiewitz, S. L. Clifasefi, J. Grow, N. Chawla, S. H. Hsu, H. A. Carroll, *et al.* "Relative Efficacy of Mindfulness-Based Relapse Prevention, Standard Relapse Prevention, and Treatment as Usual for Substance Use Disorders: A Randomized Clinical Trial." *JAMA Psychiatry* (2014).

13.   L. Festinger. "Cognitive Dissonance." *Scientific American* 207, no. 4 (1962): 93–107.

14.   R. A. Cormier. "Predicting Treatment Outcome in Chemically Dependent Women: A Test of Marlatt and Gordon's Relapse Model." University of Windsor, 2000.

15.   M. A. Walton, F. G. Castro, and E. H. Barrington. "The Role of Attributions in Abstinence, Lapse, and Relapse Following Substance Abuse Treatment." *Addict Behav* 19, no. 3 (1994): 319–31.

16.   I am forever grateful for this phrase, taught to me in a modified form by one of the wisest minds in addiction therapy, Thomas Butcher, PhD.

17.   G. Marlatt. "Surfing the Urge." Inquiring Mind, https://www.inquiringmind.com/article/2602_w_marlatt-interview-with-g-alan-marlatt-surfing-the-urge/.

Appendix A:
Description and Purpose
of Different Group Types

Process Group

During all stages of treatment, clients report that one of the most valuable experiences is Process Group. Process Group is a here and now, emotions-based group therapy. Clients should be discouraged from giving advice, engaging in long soliloquies, extensive storytelling, and attempts at caretaking the feelings of other members. The therapist does not dictate workflow the majority of time, especially not at first. Process Group does not work on specific treatment assignments. Clients are encouraged to bring emotional conflict and interpersonal issues within the treatment setting as well as issues from their past into Process Group. The central goal of Process Group is learning healthy interpersonal connection and shared empathy.

The sequence of events in Process Group is:
- A mindfulness or centering exercise at the start of group.
- The leader starts with silence and lets the group anxiety determine who will speak.
- At times, the leader will encourage a client to bring issues to group.
- Once per week (or more often if necessary) the "Guidelines and Rules for Process Group" are read aloud.

Process Group begins with a mindfulness practice or centering exercise. The group leader can choose from several alternatives for the centering exercise. Mindfulness helps every participant become present mentally and emotionally, aligned to the work of psychotherapy. From time to time, it may be helpful to have each member go through a brief check-in process. Here, each member gives a brief update about his or her recovery. During check-in, he or she may bid for "time" in group to talk about a feeling, incident, or experience that has emotional issues attached to it. The group's leader prioritizes the bids for time and asks one client to start off the group process with his or her issue. Except in extraordinary circumstances, clients do not read or ask for feedback on written assignments. Such work is deferred to Assignment Group. Advice giving is strongly discouraged during the group because it diverges the Group Process, no matter how well intentioned it is. The leader regularly asks the members "What is happening in this group right now?" This helps all group members focus on feelings, interpersonal attachment states, unspoken agendas, and so on.

Clients are encouraged to express feelings, current inner struggles, issues from the past that create guilt and shame, past and present relationship problems, and struggles they are having with recovery. Because healthy attachment is a critical element of recovery (and one that is often severely damaged by addiction) clients are encouraged to relate emotionally to each other and to the group content. In Process Group, courage is defined as "allowing yourself to feel and share that feeling with others." The therapist guides with a few, carefully chosen interventions. When a client asks for help, the most common therapist response is "What does the group think?" The group therapist, like the other members, should avoid giving advice. When a client displays deep emotions, a golden opportunity arises for emotional attachment. Once the feeling has been expressed to its fullest, the therapist encourages emotional attachment through a phrase such as "Is this touching off feelings in someone else?" In a safe group , others share nuanced emotional reactions to similar events in their own lives. Through this process, a central theme develops. When a good portion of members share emotionally, then and only then does the therapist encapsulate group process into an overall theme. This most often occurs at the end of a Process Group.

If a given client's issue is complete, and his or her work has not spun off a deepening group process, the therapist gently moves on to the next individual who has bid for time. When it is unclear as to the first client's sense of emotional completion, the therapist might often query that individual, stating, "Do you feel complete with this issue?" This queries the first client's status, marks the end of his time, and opens the door for the next person to work. It is most often best for the leader to then go silent, allowing group anxiety to select the next client to work.

Safety and confidentiality are the two key elements of an effective Process Group. Once per week, a relatively new member of the group reads the rules for Process Group to all members. This can be done at any appropriate time during the group but should be accomplished from time to time to reinforce group structure. A copy of the Rules for Process Group appears in Appendix B.

Assignment Group

In contrast to Process Group, Assignment Group is less organic and more structured. It has a planned course for clients, who present previously assigned assignments. It is important to avoid mixing process elements into Assignment Group. This dilutes the effect of each group type and confuses clients. Every assignment facilitates RecoveryMind thinking. Examples of potential assignment presentations are: reading of a prepared "alcohol or other drug use history"; a letter requested from a family member that is read in group; presentation of a continuing care plan for group feedback; or a prepared list of negative addictive behaviors, related consequences, and benefits of staying sober.

Presenting these assignments frequently brings a deep sharing not unlike that in Process Group. If this occurs, the therapist should allow a brief digression into process-oriented psychotherapy. The Assignment Group therapist may also suggest that the evoked issue be carried into Process Group. Assignments are presented in a group setting for multiple reasons. The first of these reasons is to correct AddictBrain thinking. Despite severely impaired self-insight, clients commonly have profound insight into the AddictBrain living inside peers. Second, reviewing assignments with others amplifies the emotional component of past events. Third, sharing past painful experiences normalizes them; in doing so, clients reduce the toxic shame produced by addiction. Fourth, the sharing experience induces a healthy interdependence that promotes continued emotional growth.

Skills Training Group

Skills Training Group replaces most of the traditional lectures that clients are subjected to in other treatment environments. Research shows that the lecture style format is ineffective at teaching usable recovery skills. Therefore, every Recovery Skill is taught using a three-phase process. The three-phase process first describes the skill, then demonstrates that skill through role-play, and then the group discusses the experience, deepening learning. At times, a group facilitator will ask participants to practice the learned skill during the next several days.

Here's a break down of each step of an example Skills Group:

- The Skills Group begins with the leader labeling and defining each skill. For example, the leader may begin by stating "Today we will be learning a new skill called: Alcohol Refusal skills. This example skill is designed to help clients develop a reflexive, stereotypical response when someone offers them a drink with alcohol in it." In a brief five-minute introduction, the leader describes why this is important and that it will inevitably occur to every individual in recovery. The leader describe the limits of this technique (e.g., "It will not be helpful if you spend your leisure time in bars"). The leader will provide an expected outcome for each client (e.g., "Each of you will learn an automatic verbal and behavioral response that fits who you are and at the same time removes you from this high-risk situation."). If available, the leader hands out written information about the current skill. In this example, the leader would provide a list of potential verbal and behavioral responses that move a client into safety when pressured to consume alcohol.

- Next, the leader will walk several participants through a role-play of the skill. In this example, one volunteer will be the recovering individual and the other may provide friendly pressure to drink. The recovering individual will try several verbal responses. The entire group would provide feedback and help the protagonist refine his or her skill.

- This process is repeated several times with different scenarios relevant to the actors. Some skills can be practiced by breaking up into several simultaneous groups, with the leader moving from group to offer guidance. Learning is enhanced by a modicum of fun, but should never be allowed to degrade into a mockery of the process. If an important process emerges, the leader can signal the group to focus on this event, discussing critical details of a given skill.

- Finally, some Recovery Skills Groups end with each participant writing down a short summary of what he or she has learned, steps to replicate the skill in the outside world, and the like. This written information then becomes part of that person's ongoing recovery plan.

Appendix B:
Guidelines and Rules for Process Group

Clients should read these guidelines before their first Process Group. Read each of these carefully. These guidelines will help you get the most out of your treatment experience. The bolded text should be read whenever a new member arrives and from time to time if no new members have joined. Remember, the group process is a strange territory for most people. A set of clear instructions ensures therapy occurs, instead of a social circle or chaos.

Guidelines

1. **Be on time to Process Group.** This minimizes distractions for everyone. Once the group begins the initial mindfulness centering exercise, you may not enter group.

2. **Stay in group once it begins.** The work done by patients in group deals with sensitive and intimate subject matter. Everyone feels uncomfortable emotions and vulnerable feelings from time to time. Therapy is easily sabotaged by interruptions. Therefore, it is imperative that you take care of all outside business (bathroom breaks, phone calls, finances, etc.) before and after groups. The only acceptable reason to leave a group during its process is a scheduled appointment. If you have such an appointment, you should notify the entire group during check-in. When you do have to leave, sit close to the door and step out quietly no more than five minutes prior to an appointment.

3. **Remain quiet when you're not sharing.** Stay attentive to the group process. Whispering to others during group is distracting and leads to others feeling disrespected. If you do whisper or make a comment to someone nearby, other group members may ask you to repeat what was said.

4. **Turn off mobile phones.** If cell phones are allowed in your center, the ringers should be turned completely off. Turn off vibration alerts, as they are often audible as well.

5. **Put down any writing instruments.** This includes pens, pencils, books, and pads of paper. The lessons of group therapy are absorbed through the emotional brain. Taking notes is counterproductive to psychotherapeutic growth in Process Group.

6. **Come prepared to share openly with the group.**

7. **Share your "here and now" feelings.** Tell the truth of what you're feeling and experiencing, rather than what you think others might want or expect you to say. Doing this will involve you taking emotional risks.

8. **Respectfully challenge one another when group agreements are not met.** Push each other to tell more detail about painful experiences and feelings about them.

9. **Resist using attacking language.** You may, from time to time, become agitated or angry. The group will help you express strong emotions without being hurtful to others.

10. **Maintain confidentiality.** Everything that is shared in Process Group should remain confidential to the group. This includes who attends and what is shared. If you choose to share your own experience in a past group with someone outside of that group, be certain to describe it without revealing details about others.

11. **Do not discuss Process Group issues outside of group.** If you do talk about what happened in a past group with other group members, report these conversations back to the group at the next session. This will ensure that the group work stays inside the group therapy process.

12. **Put feelings and thoughts into words rather than actions.**

13. **Take emotional risks and be vulnerable.** Bring painful issues and problems to the group. Take risks becoming emotionally vulnerable with fellow members. You may never have an opportunity like this ever again in your life, so seize the moment and make the most you can about this unique experience.

14. **Sit upright in your chair with feet and four chair legs on the floor**. Your body posture communicates to others about your attitude towards the group and its content. Slouching or turning sideways in your chair communicates a message to the group. Other members will ask you to verbalize postures so they may all learn about your unconscious intent.

Safety Rules

1. Safety rules must not be violated in Process Group.
2. No group member should exhibit physical violence toward other people or objects. This includes throwing objects and threatening postures. If you have concerns about your anger escalating into violence, let a staff member know before the group begins.

3. No group member should engage in verbal attacks on other patients or staff. Verbal expressions of violence including cursing, name-calling or yelling at others destroys the safety of Process Group. To heal in recovery, you must learn to respect others. Verbal aggression can cause just as much emotional harm as physical aggression and will not be tolerated.

4. Any patient who is intoxicated or otherwise impaired will be asked to leave. Individuals who are actively using are disruptive to group process.

Appendix C:
Recovery Support Services

RecoveryMind Training focuses on the treatment of addiction disorders. This does not mean that other types of care are not essential to help someone to even get to a place in life where recovery is possible. This is where Recovery Support Services come in. Treatment providers should consider Recovery Support Services as a prerequisite for recovery, not an add-on that the care team comes up with in the latter part of a sequence of treatment.

Many Recovery Support Services must be addressed first; examples include safe housing, attention to emergent medical conditions, and stabilization of psychiatric illnesses. The list below is not exhaustive but can be considered a start. A checklist that scans for needed Recovery Support Services should be part of all initial assessments.

Transportation
- Needs transportation services for treatment, therapy, work, or school access or access to religious services.
- Needs driver's license or other governmental identification.
- Needs help accessing public transportation.
- Needs help repairing an automobile for work or to access treatment.
- Requires specialty transportation due to physical mobility issues.

Medical and Psychiatric Care
- Has a disease that requires significant chronic care and requires ongoing support to maintain that care.
- Has an illness that requires expensive medication or surgical intervention and cannot afford such care.

- Needs training to improve medical self-care.
- Needs help finding a physician.
- Needs routine follow up with a physician's office or medical clinic.
- Needs help finding ongoing psychiatric care that supports addiction recovery.
- Needs a referral for psychiatric care.
- Needs referral to therapy.
- Needs referral for physical or sexual abuse recovery.
- Needs referral for treatment of Post-Traumatic Stress Disorder.

Occupational

- Needs help finding employment.
- Needs work skills training.
- Needs training services to improve employability.
- Has legal issues that complicate employment.

Child and Elder Care and Partner Services

- Needs child or elder care to improve access to treatment, employment, or educational services.
- Requires additional training in child or elder care.
- Needs parenting skills training.
- Needs marital assistance.

Legal

- Needs help managing probation or parole.
- Needs legal advice or counsel.
- Needs access to affordable legal aid.
- Needs legal assistance with divorce.
- Needs legal assistance with child or elder custody.

Education

- Needs language skills training.
- Needs literacy training.
- Needs a GED.
- Needs additional vocational training.
- Needs testing to determine work skills and work placement.

- Needs additional education or vocational training in an environment that is recovery friendly.

Housing and Self-Care

- Needs a home or temporary place to live.
- Needs proper clothing and footwear.
- Has a home but is in danger of losing it and needs housing assistance.
- Has a place to live but needs help making it safe from physical or sexual violence.
- Has a place to live but needs help making it safe from substance use.
- Needs a living environment that is not only safe from substance use but one that directly promotes recovery.

Spiritual

- Needs help finding spiritual or religious services.
- Needs help managing addiction as it relates to his or he faith.

Several excellent resources are helpful with understanding the role of Recovery Support Services in recovery and may help refine this list:

- SAMHSA: https://www.samhsa.gov/recovery
- Faces and Voices of Recovery: https://facesandvoicesofrecovery.org/resources/